APR   98

Modeling
Healthy
Behavior

Actions and Attitudes
in Schools

Judy C. Berryman, MA
and
Kathryn W. Breighner

ETR ASSOCIATES
Santa Cruz, California
1994

ETR Associates (Education, Training and Research) is a nonprofit organization committed to fostering the health, well-being and cultural diversity of individuals, families, schools and communities. The publishing program of ETR Associates provides books and materials that empower young people and adults with the skills to make positive health choices. We invite health professionals to learn more about our high-quality publishing, training and research programs by contacting us at P.O. Box 1830, Santa Cruz, CA 95061-1830.

About the Authors

Judy C. Berryman, MA, is the executive director of the Greater Battle Creek Healthy Lifestyles Project in Battle Creek, Michigan. The project is a school-based health promotion and education project for school staff, students and parents. She has eight years experience as an educator, trainer, lecturer and consultant in the areas of school worksite wellness, community collaboration for healthy children, and comprehensive health education. She has also served as president of the Michigan School Health Association.

Kathryn W. Breighner is a health education consultant from Harbor Springs, Michigan. She is coauthor of *I Am Amazing,* a program promoting health, safety and self-esteem. She serves as chair of the American School Health Association's council on early childhood health education and services and is a consultant with the Healthy Lifestyles Project, Battle Creek, Michigan.

© 1994 by ETR Associates. All rights reserved.

Published by ETR Associates, P.O. Box 1830, Santa Cruz, California 95061-1830

Printed in the United States of America
10 9 8 7 6 5 4 3 2 1

Cover design by Daniel Cook
Text design by Ann Smiley

Title No. H336

Library of Congress Cataloging-in-Publication Data

Berryman, Judy C.
    Modeling healthy behavior : actions and attitudes in schools / Judy C. Berryman and Kathryn W. Breighner.
       p. cm.
     1. Health education—United States. 2. Students—Health and hygiene—United States. 3. Physical fitness for children—United States. I. Breighner, Kathryn W. II. Title.
LB1588.U6B47   1994
371.7'1—dc20   93-4787

Contents

Introduction

The health issues facing children today are dramatically different from those of a few decades ago. Not too long ago, communicable diseases that were unpredictable and unavoidable were the most prevalent causes of concern.

Today, however, many of the threats to children's health and well-being are known to be linked to specific behaviors. Unhealthy eating habits, inadequate physical activity, substance use (including tobacco, alcohol and other drugs) and early sexual activity—all of these behaviors not only pose a major threat to children's health, but increase the possibility that children will develop chronic problems when they reach adulthood.

These kinds of health risks are not healed by an injection or prescription. Greater emphasis on health promotion and prevention is needed. Clearly, children in our society receive mixed messages about health. For example, we teach children that smoking is harmful; but cigarettes are widely available, and smoking is still allowed in many public places.

Yet, we do have some control over our immediate social environment and over our own behavior when it comes to health-related activities. Adults, especially parents and educators, act as models in children's lives. As models, we are highly influential in creating the health habits that will be prevalent in the next generation of adults. We need to increase our awareness of this role and its influence on children.

Parents and educators can work together to model healthy behaviors, but we need to be aware of our own health habits, values and beliefs. A look at our own foundations gives us an idea of the behaviors and beliefs we sometimes unwittingly demonstrate. To be able to provide the best possible modeling, we may need to bolster a shaky foundation.

This book is designed to help you examine your foundation. It was written especially for educators and, through them, for parents. The health beliefs, attitudes and practices of both educators and parents are powerful models for children's behavior.

Note: For simplicity, we have chosen to use the term *parents* throughout this book to refer to children's primary caregivers, although we are well aware of the diversity of family structures in today's society. We have used the term to refer to the generic role of a parent, and thus to whomever is filling that role.

How to Use This Book

The chapters in this book focus on vital health issues for children. Each chapter provides background information on the topic, then asks you to use self-assessments to reflect on your own attitudes, beliefs and actions. As you work through the self-assessments, be honest with yourself. You don't need to write out the answers to these questions. Just think of an honest answer and try to imagine how your behaviors and habits are observed by your students and the other people in your life.

The chapters also contain suggestions for connecting with families, with suggested self-assessments for parents. Appendix B contains sample letters on each topic, which can be sent home to families. Parents and other family members can do their own self-assessments to help them reflect on what they may be communicating and modeling to their children, intentionally or unintentionally.

The self-assessments can be used in a variety of ways. They might be used simply to open a dialogue on the potentially sensitive subject of what we model for children. For example, some of the self-assessment questions might be good discussion material for a school staff meeting or a parent/teacher gathering. Providing some of this information to the school board so members can inspect their own foundation might also be helpful.

Whether you are a parent or an educator, knowing what kinds of behaviors are modeled in both the home and the school can help you with your own modeling. As parents read the self-assessment questions in the chapter on fitness, some of which focus on the value of promoting lifetime skills such as running, walking, skiing or swimming, they may be encouraged to talk to the school about the kinds of skills being taught. Similarly, self-assessment questions for parents that ask if children eat breakfast or get enough sleep may prompt educators, who know that well-fed and well-rested children perform better in the classroom, to ask these same questions of their students' families.

The information in each chapter may be relevant across a number of health issues. For example, some of the questions you ask yourself in the self-esteem assessments may also apply to discussions about stress. Some actions, such as complimenting children as they complete tasks, not only help build self-esteem but also reduce stress.

The area of communication also applies to many different health issues. Communication skills are modeled daily by educators, parents and other adults. Communication is not only important in daily life and relationships, it also assists in building self-esteem and reducing stress.

The book begins with a discussion in Chapter 1 of why models matter and why educators and parents need to become partners in assessing the messages they give children. It also considers some of the silent messages we convey to children and the relationships we have with others.

Chapter 2 looks at the development of self-esteem. The self-assessments in this chapter can serve as guides to modeling behavior that promotes children's self-esteem.

Chapter 3 discusses children's eating habits and the messages about food that are conveyed to children in their school and home environments. It explores feelings and beliefs about food, along with some of the unhealthy behaviors and serious problems such as eating disorders that develop as a result of these feelings. The chapter includes suggestions for creating positive, healthy attitudes toward food and developing healthful eating patterns.

Ways of assessing how well your school and family environments support regular exercise and the modeling of physical fitness are presented in Chapter 4. Self-assessment tools offer suggestions for how to incorporate exercise and fitness into children's everyday life—both inside and outside the classroom.

In Chapter 5, the issue of substance use is discussed. Many children are apt to encounter greater inconsistencies between what is taught and what is modeled in this area than in other areas. This chapter is designed to help you uncover hidden messages children may be receiving, to offer support and resources for treating substance use problems, and to give you ideas for positive modeling and prevention.

Chapter 6 covers the topic of stress. The chapter's self-assessments provide ways to examine your own stress levels. The chapter also identifies positive ways of coping with everyday stressors in our lives—and ways to model these coping techniques for children.

Chapter 7 guides you through the contemplation of your own attitudes and actions relating to health habits, injury prevention and safety and the evaluation of the impact they might have on children.

As you work through the book, think of the assessments as a journey of self-exploration. In writing this book, we were surprised to find that the two of us, who considered ourselves attuned to health education issues, had some shaky areas of our own. You may also discover some new things about the social environment at school or at home that affect what is modeled for children.

Reflecting on your own attitudes and behaviors and trying to imagine the way others perceive you can be difficult. But as you do so, you'll see the positive impact you can have as you expand your storehouse of skills for modeling healthy behaviors. Remember, there is no single "right" way to behave. The goal of these assessments is to increase your sensitivity about the impact of modeled behavior on children. This knowledge can help guide your future actions. Only through careful inspection of our own health behaviors and how these behaviors are modeled for children will we begin to provide today's young people with the proper foundation for long, healthy lives.

The authors wish to thank the W.K. Kellogg Foundation, Battle Creek, Michigan, for their committment to health and health education.

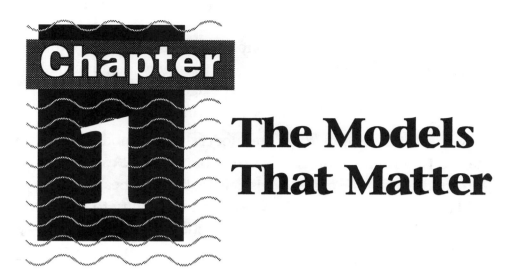

Chapter 1
The Models That Matter

TODAY'S MODELS CONTRIBUTE to the development of tomorrow's healthy adults. The health habits adults "model" affect many of the health behaviors children learn. Modeling refers to habits or behaviors that are actually demonstrated. For example, adults may tell children to wear their safety belts but then forget to fasten their own. Children hear the words, but their observation of the actions has more impact.

Children's lives are filled with models—parents, teachers, family members, next-door neighbors, school administrators, school nurses, clergy and many others. Beyond the adults who are part of children's everyday lives are other models. The media—newspapers, magazines, television and movies—present powerful models that shape behavior, influencing what we eat or drink, what we drive, what we buy.

Celebrities are powerful models, too. Athletes who demonstrate commitment to their sports through hard work and sound nutrition may be forceful teachers for young athletes. However, celebrities may not always model healthy behaviors.

Actors or others who are sexually promiscuous do not offer healthy models for safer sexual behavior. Popular songs by rock music groups may model the use of drugs or alcohol. Television programs that portray only thin teenagers suggest that fat teenagers are abnormal. Cigarette ads often feature glamorous and exciting lifestyles. Liquor commercials often display lush and elegant settings.

Everywhere children look, there are models. A role model can be someone special whom children look up to, but a model can also be anyone in children's lives. These models help instill good health habits as well as bad ones. While adults may not have the ability to change the attitudes and beliefs fostered by external models such as the media, they can examine their own lives to see what kinds of messages they are delivering to the children in their care.

Just Like Dominoes

Everything we do affects others around us. Each and every day, the actions we take and the words we say are observed and perhaps, learned, by others. We are like dominoes—each of our actions creates a wave of reaction. A happy, cheerful educator can inspire a happy, cheerful classroom. An unhappy, critical educator may prompt children to feel unsure of themselves.

Many schools have addressed the issues of health education in the past few years, and many have added health education curricula. But the curriculum areas—nutrition, fitness, health and safety, stress, self-esteem, substance use—may be modeled in an entirely different fashion than they are taught.

This conflict between teaching and practice confuses children. Children trust the adults around them and strive to act as these adults do. The actions we model are critical to establishing patterns of healthy behaviors, attitudes, values and beliefs in children.

Studies show that most of the behaviors we exhibit as adults we learned at young ages. If these behaviors include, for example, eating nutritionally poor foods, ignoring safety rules and being critical of others, then our children may internalize and pass on to their children the same behaviors.

What if these same children could watch adults eat healthy foods, exercise regularly, offer compliments for good performance, encourage participation, communicate with others and treat everyone with respect? What kinds of behaviors would these children model when they reach adulthood?

The most important risk factors for health problems in adulthood stem from behaviors learned while young. Childhood is the prime time for the development of healthy behaviors. For example, it is much easier to prevent the use of alcohol and other drugs than to intervene once these habits are in place.

The same holds true for healthy behaviors involving fitness, diet and hygiene. Children who enjoy biking, skiing or walking with their families and who eat balanced meals low in salt and fat will adopt these health habits as part of their daily lives. Children who have never exercised outside physical education classes and who have a diet of fast foods will find it difficult to adopt healthier lifestyles.

The earlier children learn and practice healthy behaviors, the more likely they are to establish these behaviors as healthy habits.

A Firm Foundation

Childhood is the perfect time to build a firm foundation for a healthy lifestyle through the promotion and maintenance of healthy behaviors. Even young children begin to show the effects of poor health habits. As much as 40 percent of children ages five to eight are obese. A poor diet and lack of exercise may contribute to higher risk of cardiovascular disease for these children as they grow older. The time to learn behaviors that will bring about healthier living is during childhood.

The American Medical Association suggests that there is an adolescent health crisis in this country. As noted in *Code Blue: Uniting for Healthier Youth,* "For the first time in the history of this country, young people are less healthy and less prepared to take their places in society than were their parents. And this is happening at a time when our society is more complex, more challenging, and more competitive than ever before" (National Commission on the Role of the School and the Community in Improving Adolescent Health, 1990).

These health behaviors have a direct link to academic performance. Students who are tired, ill, poorly nourished or live in households where there is little support and encouragement will not be in a position to learn at school.

As Dr. Michael McGinnis, director of the Office of Disease Prevention and Health Promotion, has said, "A student who is not healthy, who suffers from an undetected vision or hearing defect, or who is impaired by drugs or alcohol, is not a student who will profit from the educational process. Likewise, an individual who has not been provided assistance in the shaping of healthy attitudes, beliefs, and habits early in life, will be more likely to suffer the consequences of reduced productivity in later years"(Cohen, 1992).

The Models We Live By

Children's beliefs, standards and values give direction to their lives, and those standards and values are modeled by those around them. Models not only teach habits and behaviors but are checkpoints along the way. Children can look to their models to check their behavior, to see if they are on track or need some assistance.

Reynold Bean (1992) observed that being able to refer to models is one of the conditions for developing high self-esteem. Models enable children to make sense of the world. The ability to refer to models to help set goals and develop values, personal standards and ideals has been called a "sense of models."

We use several different types of models to make sense of the world. *Human models* include real people—such as parents or teachers—and fictional characters—perhaps a hero in a book or a character in a television program. *Philosophical models* include ideas, values and beliefs that guide behavior. *Operational models* are mental constructs learned through repetitive behavior, such as covering the mouth when yawning or shaking hands when greeting someone.

Children with a high sense of models are able to refer to human, philosophical and operational models that help them make sense of the world and their place within it. Using these reference points helps these children gain satisfaction from setting goals and create personal standards and ideals.

What does all of this mean for children's health? In order to develop healthy behaviors, children need to have adults in their lives *(human models)* who embody characteristics of a healthy lifestyle that children can emulate. When *philosophical models* are positive health-related beliefs or principles, they help children develop healthy lifestyles. The *operational models* children then develop can give them a set of concrete healthy behaviors to practice in their everyday lives.

Educators and Parents as Partners

As educators, we must examine our own habits, beliefs and attitudes, since these are the habits we model for the children in our lives. We must be aware that we model these habits and beliefs each and every day, and this modeling is a powerful lesson.

The concept of modeling in the school setting is not new. Listen to

Horace Mann in *On the Art of Teaching:*

> The school and its playground, next to the family table, are the places where the selfish propensities come into most direct collision with social duties. Here, then a right direction should be given to the growing mind. The surrounding influences which are incorporated into its new thoughts and feelings, and make part of their substance are too minute and subtle to be received in masses like nourishment; they are rather imbibed into the system unconsciously by every act of respiration, and are constantly insinuating themselves into it through all the avenues of the senses. If, then, the manners of the teacher are to be imitated by his pupils, if he is the glass at which they 'do dress themselves,' how strong is the necessity that he should understand those nameless and innumerable practices in regard to deportment, dress, conversation, and all personal habits that constitute the difference between a gentleman and a clown.

When did Mr. Mann make this observation? In 1840!

Educators may not be aware of the health habits they model to children. Schools, for example, might place little emphasis on physical education, serve vending machine lunches that are nutritionally weak, and do little to encourage teachers to be fit and healthy. Students then see that daily exercise, good food and fitness are not values promoted by the school. Educators may not eat the school lunch, suggesting to students that these lunches are not desirable or appropriate for adults, or they may demonstrate excessive concern about weight, communicating to children that being thin at all costs is important.

Educators model habits and beliefs for a good portion of the student's day. Educators need to know how important they are in instilling healthy habits in their students. They also can play an important role in educating parents and families.

Open lines of communication with families not only educate parents and other family members, but allow for the sharing of valuable information about children. Newsletters about nutrition, safety, self-esteem or fitness can be sent home.

Parents have a responsibility not only to be good models, but also to know what is happening in the school. If parents are taking steps to increase children's self-esteem but the school counteracts those steps through attitudes or actions that discourage children, the parents' task is much more difficult.

Parents should know what kinds of modeling are taking place in school. Talking to an educator or school administrator can provide answers; it also provides many opportunities to communicate. Parents may also be able to observe or participate in children's classrooms. The parent's role in the modeling that takes place in school is just as important as the modeling that takes place at home.

Parents and educators who work together as partners in the modeling of healthy behaviors can be much more successful in raising happy, healthy children. Just knowing that we have the ability to shape children's future health habits is like opening a door. This knowledge makes it much easier for us to look at what we do and say, and to change our habits, if we need to and if we can, for our children.

Silent Messages

Look around you in a group setting. Can you tell how people are feeling based on their body language and appearance? A colleague drags his feet and his shoulders sag as he walks. Is he happy and full of energy? Probably not. He is probably feeling tired, sad or sick. Another colleague might be sitting upright at a desk, eyes alert, leaning forward to listen. She is engaged and energetic. Yet another colleague is fidgeting, shifting in his seat and nervously twisting paper clips. Body language gives us many clues to a person's state of mind.

Think about a classroom where the teacher comes in with droopy eyes and a sad face. She does not say a word, yet the students know how this teacher is feeling. Body language tells others how we are feeling in clear and expressive ways. The way we look can indicate whether we are happy, sad, tired, bored, ill or angry.

Communicating with children involves more than just words. Often how we act and how we look may be very different from our words. A child may be talking about his day at school while we unload the dishwasher, fix dinner and make a grocery list. We interject with an occasional "That's nice" while the child is talking, but we are not really listening, and we do not fool the child.

Habits such as twisting hair, cracking knuckles, yawning or bouncing a leg are nonverbal cues. Teachers can easily spot students who are not focused. Such students might be looking out the window or doodling on their note pads.

The reverse is also true. Students can tell by a teacher's yawning or pacing that their discussion and comments are not really being heard. Tone of voice also indicates feelings. The educator may say, "Let's open our books and read this together," in a tone that suggests cooperation, excitement, boredom, anger, fatigue or frustration. The meaning of the words is influenced by the tone.

Self-Assessment: Silent Messages at School

Body language and tone of voice often result in the modeling of mixed messages, and students do not know which message to believe—the one that is stated or the one that is modeled. Think about the types of nonverbal communication you use daily. For example, do you think children can tell if you are angry or tired before you've said a word? If the answer is yes, then your nonverbal cues have given you away. In this first self-assessment, you'll reflect on your nonverbal communication with others.

As an educator, do you:

■ Notice your body language when you are happy?

- Notice your body language when you are sad/angry/tired?

- Think you can guess how a colleague feels by how she or he looks?

- Think your students know how you are feeling by how you look?

- Truly listen when your students are talking?

- Think your students know you listen when they talk?

- Make eye contact when you talk and listen?

- Take part in extra activities with your students (such as helping with special projects or walking with them during lunch hour)?

- Shake hands when you meet someone?

- Easily give hugs or pats on the back?

- Know how your students feel by their actions?

- Notice your students' body language as they try to get your attention?

- Know how to acknowledge students' accomplishments without saying a word?

Relating to Others: Social Well-Being

A relationship is any kind of interaction that takes place between people. Relationships vary from the casual, with store clerks, to the more formal, with colleagues and employers, to the more intimate, with family and friends.

Children learn about relationships from the people around them. Watching the adults around them react to and with others offers children many informal lessons about relationships. They learn about relationships through this observation of adults, as well as through observation of other children interacting with those around them.

Family Connection: Considerations for Parents

Parents can also explore how aware they are of their own body language when they interact with their children. The following self-assessment for parents provides a means of reflecting on how they may use silent messages—intentionally or not—and how these messages might affect their communication with their children.

Self-Assessment: Silent Messages at Home

As a parent, do you:

- Really listen when others speak?
- Make eye contact when talking?
- Take care not to express disappointment or frustration by the look on your face when a child misses the basket in the championship basketball game or comes in wet after being caught in a sudden rainstorm?
- Hug and kiss your children often?
- Know how children are feeling by how they look and act?
- Respond to children's body language, not just their words?
- Listen to the tone of your voice when you speak?

Watch Out For...

- Body language that sends a different message than your words (for example, saying things are fine when your expression clearly shows you're angry or unhappy).

Home and classroom environments that are open, supportive and nurturing help children develop a sense of self, security, belonging, respect and worth. These environments allow children to learn the social and personal skills needed for relationships with those around them.

Adults can find many ways to show they believe relationships are important. Spending time with family and friends, talking to the clerk in the store, taking care of an elderly parent or packing special notes in a child's lunch box are all ways to show that relationships are valued.

Adults should model healthy social relationships for children. Without these models, children will have a more difficult time forming relationships with peers or with the adults in their lives. Educators who draw children into their lives with their affection, compassion, concern and laughter can teach students the value of relationships. Children need to see working relationships throughout the day.

Not all relationships are productive ones. We may find that some people in our lives are annoying or burdensome. But this is also a reality that children must learn to work with. Relationships may come and go. We may have friends we see only during the summer or family we visit just once a year, yet these relationships are still a part of us.

Some children easily make friends. They move with ease from one group of children to another. Their circle of friends is wide and varied. Other children find relationships much more difficult. They may not feel comfortable playing on the playground with a large group of children or even talking to others in the locker room.

Some children are naturally less outgoing than others. But some children may not have been exposed to the modeling of healthy social relationships, or they may lack the appropriate social skills, communication skills and self-esteem needed to establish a relationship. The skills needed to build relationships begin to develop at an early age and are refined and fine-tuned throughout life.

Self-Assessment: Modeling Relationships at School

Think about the relationships you have in your own life as well as your relationships with students. This self-assessment will help you examine your relationships and how they are modeled to children. Remember that there are many different styles of communicating with others. Not everyone is an extrovert. The important thing is to do what's comfortable for you, become more aware of what your actions tell your students, and see that there are things you can do to enhance your students' social well-being.

As an educator, do you:

- Consider yourself a good friend?

- Enjoy time with friends and family?

- Keep in touch with friends by mail or phone?

- Enjoy relationships with your colleagues and your students?

- Think your students consider you a friend?

- Include parent volunteers as part of the relationships in your classroom?

- Work at building relationships with students' families?

- Let students see you interact with other adults?

- Bring other adults into the classroom to let them interact with students?

- Trust your relationships with others?

- Observe relationships among students?

- Reach out to students who need a friend?

- Communicate honestly with students?

- Encourage students to seek or strengthen relationships?

- Talk to parents about unhealthy relationships you see developing at school?

- Use group activities to encourage communication among students?

Family Connection: Considerations for Parents

Parents' social relationships are observed daily as models by children. Parents need to be aware of the connections between their feelings about relationships and their children's relationships with others. The following self-assessment can help parents look at what their actions tell their children about relationships.

Self-Assessment: Modeling Relationships at Home

As a parent, do you:

- Think your relationships with friends and family are important?
- Get together with family members and invite friends to your home?
- Let children see that adults have good friends, too?
- Let children develop relationships with your friends?
- Help children make friends?
- Approve of your children's friends?
- Let children make decisions about their friends?
- Think your children are good friends to others?
- Think your children see you as a friend?
- Encourage relationships between children and other family members?
- Let children take part in after-school activities both at school and away from school?
- Help out at school so your children can see you relate to other children?
- Think that your children's friends like coming to your home?
- Let children see you relate to others in different settings (work, home, school, social, etc.)?

Watch Out For...

- Criticizing children's friends.
- Criticizing children for their choices in friends.

Chapter

2 Feeling Good: Personal and Social Well-Being

DEVELOPING A HEALTHY LIFESTYLE involves more than just learning a set of concrete behaviors such as crossing the street safely or exercising to keep fit. What does it mean to have a healthy lifestyle? A healthy lifestyle is a set of health-enhancing behaviors that are shaped by internally consistent values, attitudes and beliefs and are influenced by external social and cultural forces.

When we talk about health, we're talking about a state of physical, mental/emotional and social well-being, and not just the absence of disease or injury. The physical, mental/emotional and social dimensions of health are closely related to each other. For instance, a substance use problem involves the drug itself, the physical and emotional characteristics of the person using the drug, and the social and cultural context where the drug is available and used.

In this chapter, we'll look at the more abstract parts of a healthy lifestyle—working toward personal and social well-being by developing high self-esteem and healthy relationships.

Self-Esteem

Simply put, self-esteem is the way we feel about ourselves. When we have high self-esteem, we are able to feel a sense of satisfaction that comes from our own inner resources.

For children, having high self-esteem means that they feel good about themselves. They feel a sense of security and are willing to explore the world. High self-esteem helps them take risks, communicate with friends, even deal with stress, set goals and make decisions. Low self-esteem may mean that children do not feel comfortable raising their hands in class, having friends, trying out for the basketball team or even choosing what they want to eat for lunch.

Clearly, raising self-esteem is important not only for the sense of mental or emotional well-being that it creates. It also is necessary for developing the ability to choose healthy behaviors and set the goal of a healthy lifestyle.

Low self-esteem has been found to be a common thread for many of the problems of children and youth. A good example is substance use. Troubled teens with few friends and an unsupportive home life may turn to alcohol or other drugs. Students who have alcoholic parents and avoid friends because they are embarrassed about their home life may become abusive or aggressive in the classroom to gain attention. Use of alcohol or other drugs may be part of an effort to gain acceptance, call attention to oneself or be different.

Conditions of Self-Esteem

According to Bean (1992), there are four important conditions or feelings children need to experience in order to have high self-esteem. People with high self-esteem experience all of these feelings frequently, in different circumstances and with a high level of intensity. People with low self-esteem have difficulty feeling one or more of the four feelings. When one or more of these feelings is missing, feeling "bad" is the result. Persistently feeling bad is a sign of low self-esteem.

A *sense of connectiveness* is the ability to gain satisfaction from the people, places or things we feel connected to. When children have a high sense of connectiveness, they feel they are a part of something, feel they are important to others, and feel comfortable with their bodies (feel connected to themselves).

A *sense of uniqueness* is the feeling that we have qualities that are special and different. When children have a high sense of uniqueness, they feel that they are valued for who they are, and they are able to respect themselves.

A *sense of power* enables us to believe in ourselves, feel competent and feel comfortable with responsibility. When children have a high sense of power, they are able to feel in control of themselves despite pressures they might experience. They feel that others can't make them do things they really don't want to do.

A *sense of models* is the ability to refer to human, philosophical and operational models to help make sense of the world. Children with a high sense of models feel confident that they can tell right from wrong and good from bad. They have consistent values and beliefs guiding their actions in different situations, have a sense of their own standards and are able to organize their environment to accomplish a task.

As teachers, our own personal self-esteem structure is part of the picture. As Bean has noted, it is simplistic to say that you can't raise another person's self-esteem unless you have high self-esteem yourself. The relationship between educators' and students' self-esteem is more complex.

Educators are more likely to support in their students the particular conditions of self-esteem that are strongest in themselves. For example, a teacher with a high sense of connectiveness feels good about close relationships with children and highly values them in the classroom. The climate for connectiveness is good in this teacher's classroom; the teacher is sensitive and compassionate. Children who come into this class with a low sense of connectiveness will benefit from being with that teacher.

If this teacher has a low sense of power, however, children who also have a low sense of power won't experience the conditions necessary for growth in that area. As a result, some children's self-esteem will improve in this classroom, while others' may not.

Self-Assessment: Your Self-Esteem Foundation

In the following self-assessment, reflect on how you feel about yourself. How do you feel about who you are and what you have accomplished? How do you project your feelings of self-worth to those around you? How you model these feelings to children not only lets them know how you feel about yourself but suggests to them that they might feel the same way.

In addition to looking at how you feel about yourself, take a look at what you do in your life to help you feel more secure and confident. The steps that you take not only help you feel better but also show others (especially children) that you care about yourself.

As you do the self-assessment, remember that there's no "perfect" self-esteem profile. Everyone has areas that are strong and areas that are more challenging for them. The goal is to learn to work well with what you have and to make changes where you can. In examining your own level of self-esteem, you'll be better able to understand how your self-esteem and students' interact to affect the learning process as well as your own feelings of comfort and satisfaction in the classroom.

As an educator, do you:

- Feel good about yourself?

- Have a support network of friends, colleagues or family?

- Feel that you have accomplished goals that are important to you?

■ Have skills you feel good about?

■ Care about the people in your life and show it?

■ Trust other people?

■ Trust yourself and the decisions you make?

■ Enjoy what you do and convey this to others?

■ Consider yourself enthusiastic?

■ Feel secure in your personal life?

■ Accept others as they are?

■ Set realistic limits for yourself?

■ Help yourself to feel your best (e.g., by eating well and exercising)?

■ Enjoy activities, such as walking, swimming or biking, that increase your self-esteem?

■ Get regular physical checkups?

■ Participate in extracurricular activities that you enjoy and let others see you doing so?

Watch Out For...

■ Being self-critical.

■ Fearing failure.

■ Always comparing yourself with others.

■ Criticizing others as a way to feel better about yourself.

Self-Assessment: Self-Esteem in the Classroom

You can do much to establish a trusting, nurturing environment in the classroom. How you act toward students—and yourself—are important modeling actions. The silent messages we model reflect concepts such as discipline, fairness and trust. Building your students' self-esteem models the value that feeling good about yourself is important. Children notice when we respect others, and repeated classroom modeling and reinforcement can help them learn to act this way themselves.

As an educator, do you:

■ Set realistic limits for your students?

■ Provide rules or guidelines for acceptable behavior?

■ Enforce rules consistently?

■ Create a trusting classroom environment?

■ Respect your students?

■ Think your students respect you?

■ Recognize the uniqueness of each of your students?

■ Encourage students to develop their special qualities?

■ Help students recognize their personal strengths?

■ Encourage students to accomplish goals for their own personal satisfaction?

■ Encourage students to spend extra time doing things they do well?

■ Encourage students to accept others as they are?

■ Compliment students on accomplishments?

■ Know which rewards work with your students?

■ Know when to arrange class rewards such as a party?

■ Encourage students to take risks and offer support when they do?

■ Recognize students with low self-esteem and find activities to help them?

■ Include parents in a team effort to build self-esteem?

■ Refer students for professional help with self-esteem when needed?

- Use a classroom curriculum on self-esteem?
- Send information on self-esteem home?
- Encourage students to participate in extracurricular activities that build personal skills?
- Encourage your school to start extracurricular activities?
- Recognize colleagues with low self-esteem?
- Regularly compliment colleagues?
- Actively encourage parents to participate in the classroom?
- Expose students to a variety of enrichment experiences such as field trips?
- Explore cultural differences such as holiday celebrations?
- Know when to call for help from a parent or aide when you're having a bad day?

Watch Out For...

- Showing favoritism.
- Comparing students to one another.
- Punishing poor performance with loss of privileges (such as recess).
- Discouraging students from trying new things because they take too much of your time.
- Criticizing students when you're having a hard day.
- Making negative comments about students to other teachers or parents.

Family Connection: Considerations for Parents

Displaying feelings of self-worth and accomplishment not only lets children know that we feel good about ourselves but shows them that they can feel the same way. This is true at home as well as in the classroom. Parents can also look at how they feel about themselves. Children are very observant, and by observing parents' everyday actions, children probably are aware of how their parents feel.

The home environment is an important component in teaching children how to feel good about themselves. When parents express positive feelings toward children, it helps children feel secure and happy and teaches them that showing these feelings is part of everyday life and of parenting. With the modeling of these feelings, parents express their hope that their children will grow up to be nurturing, caring parents as well.

Parents can do much to establish the building blocks for high esteem in their children. The successes that children find in their daily lives can be important steps to helping them grow up to be happy, secure adults.

Parents with high self-esteem can model this for children. For example, letting children feel that they are a part of the family with duties and responsibilities, just like the adults, helps them not only to feel responsible, but to be active participants in the family process. Encouraging family activities may help children learn that family activities are fun while boosting their self-esteem when they've mastered ice skating or created a sand castle.

The following self-assessment asks parents to look at the self-esteem building opportunities they have with their children.

Self-Assessment: Self-Esteem at Home
Your Own Self-Esteem

As a parent, do you:

- Feel good about who you are?
- Feel secure in your daily life?
- Enjoy your role as parent?
- Have a supportive spouse, partner, family or friends?
- Feel appreciated?
- Feel good about the goals you have met?
- Think that your children see you as happy and secure?
- Share your successes with children?

(continued)

Modeling Self-Esteem

As a parent, do you:

- Notice children's special qualities?
- Feel proud of your children?
- Focus on children's strengths?
- Show sincere interest in what children do?
- Act as if you expect children to succeed?
- Provide positive feedback?
- Listen carefully to children?
- Know what children expect and want?
- Expect actions that are consistent with children's abilities and desires?
- Let children know what you expect?
- Spend quiet time with children to talk and share feelings?
- Appreciate children and show it?

Building Self-Esteem

As a parent, do you:

- Know when children are feeling low self-esteem?
- Know how to boost children's self-esteem?
- Let children succeed on their own, even though you could do it faster or better?
- Focus on the joys of playing a game or sport rather than winning or being perfect?
- Give children household chores or duties?
- Think your children are responsible family members?
- Compliment children on what they do?
- Help children learn new skills and develop new interests?
- Let children take part in after-school activities that help them improve their skills and social abilities?
- Let children take part in after-school activities that they like?
- Spend time together as a family to learn new skills or just have fun?
- Take time to be part of children's activities?
- Think your children see that you are interested in their lives?
- Enjoy your own activities and let children see this?
- Encourage children to be independent?
- Sometimes help arrange events so that children can be successful?
- Stay in touch with the school?
- Talk to teachers about ways to increase children's self-esteem?
- Know what kind of skills or curricula your children's teachers use to build self-esteem?

(continued)

Watch Out For...
- Feeling guilty.
- Talking often about failures in front of children.
- Easily getting upset when criticized.
- Comparing yourself to others.
- Making sarcastic remarks to children.
- Easily getting angry.
- Making critical remarks (for example, "Why did you do that? That was a stupid thing to do.").
- Comparing one child to another.
- Telling children, "You can't do that. You don't know how."
- Planning so much for children to do that they don't have time to relax.
- Focusing too much on winning or performing perfectly.

Values and Beliefs

The standards, values and beliefs that we hold give shape and direction to our lives. How we act, think, make decisions, feel about ourselves and treat others are derived from personal values, ideals, goals and beliefs that come largely from our family, friends and school.

Values come in many forms. They may be religious, social, personal or family oriented, and decisions often are made consistent with what we believe. Values a school or family might teach include respect for authority, respect for others, and respect for the unique qualities of each of us. Schools and families can foster a healthy self-concept, a desire to learn and the freedom to experiment.

The choices students make are often connected to their values. Children who taunt other children because they wear glasses may have values that do not include respect for others. Children who help other children with their class work may possess values that include helping and respecting others.

A family that does not value education might raise children who are not high academic achievers. Such students may seek out friends with similar values. These students may be just as bright as their academically successful peers, but their classroom performance reflects the values established by their family and friends. On the other hand, families who feel that education is essential, relish learning, encourage reading and instill good work habits are teaching children that education is a value that is important.

Children who come to school feeling they are stupid, ugly, unloved or unworthy usually feel this way because the people around them have suggested that these beliefs are true. Positive beliefs let children feel happy, loved, unique, and good about themselves. Educators play an important role in providing positive reinforcement that all children are unique, special and valued. This reinforcement is particularly critical for those children who do not get such reinforcement at home.

Locus of Control

Locus of control relates to our sense of control of our behavior. Do we take responsibility for our behavior (internal locus of control), or do we attribute it to other sources (external locus of control)?

Individuals with an internal locus of control believe that the control is within themselves. Failing to turn in homework or being late for the dentist is due to actions we take. People with an external locus of control place the blame on other sources. The homework was late because the parent forgot to wake up the child early. The dentist appointment was hard to get to because the phone kept ringing and the clock was slow. Children need to feel that they are in control and that their behavior is guided by their actions, not others'.

Some events *are* beyond students' control. A student may be late for school because the parent did not leave home in time. Children need to understand that some actions are out of their control and learn not to feel guilty about being in situations where they are blameless.

Children who have values consistent with an internal locus of control feel in control and are willing to make choices and decisions to accomplish their goals. Growing up with a solid foundation of values that clearly sets parameters for behavior helps children feel confident in the ability to make something good of their lives and to have an impact on the lives of others. Children with this kind of foundation have a high sense of models. Such children are less likely to develop substance use problems or other behavioral difficulties stemming from peer pressure.

Self-Assessment: Your Values and Beliefs

Values and beliefs are important concepts to model. Those who teach these concepts are helping to establish patterns that may last a lifetime. As you go through this self-assessment, think about how you feel, act out and model concepts such as honesty or taking responsibility for your actions. Think about the values and beliefs that you possess and consider how these are modeled in daily life. It is sobering to remember that children are learning that these are beliefs they should possess as well.

As an educator, do you:

- Consider yourself a compassionate person?
- Remember your childhood heroes/heroines? What were the attributes you admired?
- Teach because you want to contribute to the next generation?
- Feel that you have many good qualities?
- Find it easy to name ten of your good qualities?
- Feel that you are an honest, fair person?
- Think that your students view you as honest and fair?
- Admit your mistakes?
- Express your feelings in appropriate ways when you are angry?
- Accept responsibility for your actions?

■ Operate from an internal locus of control?

■ Volunteer time to help organizations or causes?

■ Feel you are tolerant of people's differences?

Self-Assessment: Modeling Values and Beliefs in the Classroom

The classroom environment offers many opportunities to model values and beliefs. A classroom based on responsibility, compassion and acceptance of people's differences demonstrates to students that these are important values to live by. In the next self-assessment, you'll consider the ways you model your values and beliefs in the classroom.

As an educator, do you:

■ Clearly outline classroom responsibilities and rules?

■ Let your students make choices that put their values to work?

■ Realize that discipline reflects your values by reinforcing fairness, honesty and acceptance of responsibility?

■ Expect your students to be responsible for their actions?

■ Treat each child fairly?

■ Encourage students to be honest, fair, caring?

■ Encourage compassion for others through projects such as making gifts for families or visiting a nursing home?

■ Encourage students and families to be community minded?

■ Think your students see you as an active person in the community?

■ Include your classroom in community projects such as planting trees or recycling?

■ Encourage discussion about the special qualities of all people and how they are valued?

- Encourage discussion about cultural diversity?
- Talk about public figures who model important values and beliefs?

Family Connection: Considerations for Parents

The values and beliefs that we possess affect how we treat and act with our children. Parents often model the very values and beliefs that were modeled to them as children. These are the values and beliefs that have become important to them. The view children have of their parents' qualities provides clues as to what their parents are modeling to them.

For example, honesty is not reinforced as a value when a parent calls in sick and then spends the day at the beach. On the other hand, the family that "adopts" another family at Thanksgiving or any other time teaches compassion in an active, modeled way, and demonstrates the value of caring for others.

The following self-assessment helps parents look at some of the ways they model their beliefs and values at home.

Self-Assessment: Modeling Values and Beliefs at Home

As a parent, do you:
- Think you are a caring, compassionate person?
- Remember your childhood heroes/heroines and talk about them with children?
- Realize how important you are in helping children become caring, honest adults?
- Think your children can name some of your good qualities?
- Talk about good qualities in your children, family and friends?
- Treat children with affection?
- Encourage children to show affection?
- Let children make choices that use their values?
- Encourage children to care for others?
- Admit mistakes to yourself and children?
- Accept responsibility for your actions?
- Discipline children fairly?
- Use discipline to reinforce family values and beliefs such as fairness, honesty or compassion?

(continued)

Modeling Healthy Behavior

- Let children know you value education?
- Give time to your children's school?
- Give to your community through volunteer efforts?
- Let children show their anger in appropriate ways, such as saying how they feel?
- Show children that anger is normal?
- Show your own anger without criticizing or making threats you do not mean?
- Talk about your feelings with children?
- Let children talk about their feelings?
- Encourage children to be responsible at home?
- Schedule family time (to read, watch a movie, go for a walk, take a vacation, enjoy a meal, etc.)?

Watch Out For...
- Modeling dishonest behavior, such as parking in a handicapped zone without a permit or keeping too much change when the grocery clerk makes a mistake.
- Making critical comments about others.
- Showing prejudice against people who are different in any way.

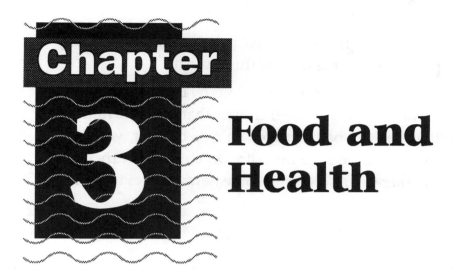

Chapter

3 Food and Health

AS THE LINKS BETWEEN DIET and health became clear, the U.S. Department of Health and Human Services issued *Dietary Guidelines for Americans*. The 1990 edition of this report made the following recommendations for changes in Americans' eating habits.

- Reduce intake of fat to less than 30 percent and intake of saturated fats to less than 10 percent of the total dietary intake.

- Increase consumption of fruits and vegetables.

- Reduce sugar intake.

- Increase consumption of whole-grain products.

- Reduce salt consumption.

- Reduce total calorie intake.

Putting these guidelines into practice may not be simple. Children and adults need a few basic building blocks in place in order to learn healthy food habits. We must learn to trust our bodies to let us know when we are hungry and when we are full. We must understand basic nutrition. We must accept the fact that people come in a variety of sizes and shapes and respect and value this diversity.

Children learn what is important to adults by listening to them and by watching them. Adults can model choices that promote nutritional health as well as healthy body images. In this chapter, you'll check your awareness of what you are modeling to children in these areas. We hope the chapter will also suggest some new avenues to explore.

Trusting the Body

Children need to learn that they can trust their bodies to let them know when they are hungry and when they are full. For infants, this is a normal process; they eat in response to body hunger cues and stop eating in response to feelings of fullness.

As children get older, external cues can start to confuse this natural ability to regulate food intake. For instance, some children get so used to eating in front of the television set that watching television—not hunger—becomes a signal to eat.

Ikeda and Naworski (1992) observed that when adults try to control the amount of food children eat, they are inadvertently telling children that they can't trust their bodies to let them know when they are hungry and when they are full and that someone else has to regulate this for them. If children are to learn to take responsibility for healthy eating habits, they must believe that they can handle this responsibility.

These authors point out that adults may find it especially difficult to let children who are overweight take control of their food intake. But attempting to control the amount of food children eat can backfire, as children who worry that they won't get enough food to satisfy their hunger may begin to seek other ways to ensure that they get what they need—such as sneaking food, hiding food or buying food when adults aren't around. As a result, children can end up eating more food rather than less.

Choosing Healthy Foods

The key to good nutrition is eating a wide variety of "nutrient-dense" foods (Ikeda and Naworski, 1992). These are foods with good nutritional value (vitamins, minerals, protein, complex carbohydrates) in relationship to their calorie value. Foods with low nutrient density have little nutritional value in relationship to their calorie value.

Within each of the basic food groups, foods can be categorized as having high nutrient density, good nutrient density or lower nutrient density. Most of the foods we eat should fall into the category of high nutrient density. Appendix A provides charts that show the nutrient density of various foods.

Foods with low nutrient density are often called *junk food*. Try to avoid the use of this term, as it implies a value judgment (which children may react to) rather than a factual assessment of the nutritional value of a food. These foods should be eaten only occasionally, not on a regular basis. However, if these foods are completely forbidden, children may begin to find them even more desirable.

Another key to developing healthy eating habits is establishing regular meals and snacks. This eating pattern keeps children's hunger satisfied, so that they are more likely to eat only the amounts they need. When children skip meals or snacks, they are more apt to overeat at the next meal because they are so hungry. When children snack constantly, they are more likely to overeat—and what they're eating is likely to have a lower nutrient density than foods served at mealtimes.

Modeling Healthy Food Habits

School staff members can have a significant influence on children's food choices and on children's perceptions of appropriate foods by what they model for children. A teacher who eats carrot sticks as a snack teaches students about healthy choices. The teacher who snacks on candy throughout the day, as students watch, is sending a message that such snacking is an acceptable way to eat.

Adults' choices of foods and eating habits affect children's beliefs and behavior. Not only do children observe what adults do and compare it with what they say; they also depend on adults to set standards and, when they are very young, to provide the foods from which to choose.

The Importance of Snacks

Snacking is an important part of a child's daily nutrition. Young children often snack several times a day, and the foods eaten as snacks make up a significant portion of the required nutrients. Yet, we often don't pay enough attention to the nutrient content of snacks. While we may try to make meals balanced and nutritious, snack time is frequently a "free time" without clearly established guidelines to follow.

Schools can significantly affect snack habits. Preschool and kindergarten children typically snack once in the morning and once in the afternoon. Older students may bring in snacks for special occasions such as birthdays or holidays. Learning good snack habits at an early age can be the beginning of a lifelong pattern of healthy eating. Schools can model healthy snacking by developing a clear, written policy regarding the nutritional value of food served at school. The following examples are from schools that were successful at this.

At a Battle Creek, Michigan, school, no "unhealthy" snacks are permitted in the classrooms or at school-sponsored events. Families are provided with a list of acceptable foods. Teachers and parents have been given a clear message from the administration, and students consistently have healthy snacks at school. Families also learn about healthy snacking from this school rule.

This school also sponsors a "fruity" Halloween party. Students come dressed as vegetables and fruits. Snacks at this event do not include cookies, cakes and candies; only fresh fruits and vegetables are served. Students, who do not go home with stomachaches from too much Halloween candy, have learned that healthy snacks taste good.

A nearby school district offers a "pumpkin prance" event at Halloween. Families—in costume—attend a one-mile walk, or prance, at local schools. Each participant receives a certificate. Pumpkin cookies, muffins and low-fat doughnuts are served with cider.

Self-Assessment: Snacking at School

Educators have many opportunities to model healthy snacking behavior during the school day. The following self-assessment can help you examine your snack habits and beliefs, both at home and at school, and look at how you model those habits to students. What types of snacks do you eat, both at home and at school? What types of snacks do students enjoy in the classroom? What are students learning from you about snacks? Consider ways you might improve your students' snack habits as well as your own.

As an educator, do you:

■ Eat healthy snacks in front of students?

■ Eat healthy snacks at home?

■ Talk about healthy snacks with students?

■ Reward students with healthy snacks?

- Know if your school has a healthy snack policy?

- Talk with other teachers about the need for healthy snacks or a healthy snack policy?

- Ask parents to bring only healthy snacks to school?

- Provide information on healthy snacks to parents?

- Make positive suggestions to parents who send unhealthy snacks to school?

- Know where to find nutritional information for parents?

- Know if your school has vending machines available to students and what kinds of foods are in these machines?

- Know what kinds of foods are sold at school-sponsored events?

- Ask school administration for juice machines rather than soda machines?

Watch Out For...

- Eating unhealthy snacks in front of students.

- Routinely keeping candy or sweets in your desk for snacks.

- Rewarding children with unhealthy snacks such as candy.

Healthy Snacks

Snack habits—and snacking—can last a lifetime. When adults model healthy snacking, children learn to make food choices that meet their daily nutritional needs.

Snacking behavior can be changed, and children can learn to enjoy healthy foods. However, it may take a few years to outgrow the desire for the old foods.

Good choices for healthy snacks include:

- fruits and vegetables

- unsweetened applesauce

- bagels, bread sticks, whole grain bread, tortillas (flour or corn)

- unsugared and low-fat cereals or cereals sweetened with fruit juice

- low-fat or nonfat milk, yogurt, frozen yogurt or cheese

- all-fruit juices (not those labeled "fruit drinks") and frozen fruit-juice bars

- dried fruits

- nuts and seeds—in moderation (Although nutrient-dense, nuts and seeds are high in fat.)

- popcorn, low-salt pretzels and rice cakes

- pudding made with nonfat milk

- matzo

Family Connection: Considerations for Parents

Some parents may not be aware of the difference between healthy and unhealthy snacks. Such parents may teach children to enjoy inappropriate snacks by offering these foods on a regular basis. Television ads that promote foods with little nutritional value and aisles of such foods in the grocery stores may contribute to parents' confusion about healthy snacks.

Young children need snacks because they cannot consume enough at one meal to sustain them until the next mealtime. Good snacks provide energy and are nutrient dense. Not only young children need snacks. Most children are hungry after school. What will they choose to eat?

A look in the home kitchen can be revealing. What kind of snacks do we make available to our children and ourselves? Do we have cookies, processed foods, high-fat chips? Do we eat the same snacks as our children? When the children are not around, what do we eat?

Parents may want to reflect on their routine snacking habits, as well as snacking behavior during special occasions or at school.

(continued)

Self-Assessment: Snacking at Home

As a parent, do you:

- Try to learn more about nutrition through reading or other sources?
- Give children several choices of healthy foods so they have chances to make decisions?
- Have family rules about snacking, such as No snacking during the hour before a meal?
- Think about healthy snacks when shopping and try to steer clear of foods high in fat and sugar?
- Ask children to help pick out healthy snacks when shopping?
- Shop with a grocery list?
- Offer healthy snacks to children?
- Know what kinds of snacks the school allows?
- Know what kinds of snacks your children eat when visiting friends?
- Take healthy snacks to school events?
- Pack healthy snacks for family outings?
- Enjoy eating healthy snacks?
- Offer sugarless gum or candies or other healthy snacks as holiday treats (for example, in Christmas stockings)?
- Hand out healthy foods or non-food items such as stickers as Halloween treats?
- Celebrate special occasions with foods low in fat or sugar such as angel food cake?
- Compliment children on their good snack habits and snack choices?

Watch Out For...

- Always offering sweets such as cookies or cake for special occasions.
- Letting children eat so many snacks that they won't eat meals.
- Letting children snack while watching TV.

Meals

The eating habits gained at mealtime are important ones. Introducing well-balanced meals to children exposes them to good foods and lets them become accustomed to these foods in their daily lives.

Breakfast is a particularly crucial meal. Children who go to school without breakfast do not perform as well as students who have eaten breakfast, as their small stomachs cannot absorb enough energy-producing food during the dinner meal to carry them through until lunch the next day. Although lunch is often the only meal teachers spend with students, good breakfasts and dinners at home show their influence in the classroom. Many schools have a breakfast program for this very reason.

Self-Assessment: Meals at School

Inadequate nutrition makes children tired, lethargic and grumpy, and these effects will show in the classroom. Children need enough fuel to get them through a busy day. If the home environment doesn't include a good breakfast and balanced and filling meals, students will have difficulty concentrating in the classroom. How aware are you of your students' nutritional patterns?

As an educator, do you:

- Talk about nutrition with your students?

- Send information on nutrition to parents and discuss it with them?

- Use an established nutrition curriculum alone or as part of a comprehensive health education curriculum?

- Know if students in your class/school are not eating breakfast?

- Refer students into a meal program for breakfast or hot lunch, if needed?

- Understand that eating balanced meals helps children be more attentive in the classroom?

- Consider having family nights where each family brings in a food of their choice from one of the food groups?

Family Connection: Considerations for Parents

Home is the setting where most habits about meals are developed. Parents may not realize that fast-food dinners and frozen or highly processed meal choices may be teaching children that these foods are what meals are all about. Children learn about balanced, nutritious meals by eating them on a daily basis.

Parents can reflect on the meal patterns at home and the kinds of modeling children see at mealtime.

Self-Assessment: Meals at Home

As a parent, do you:

- Plan balanced meals on a regular basis?
- Eat only a little of fast foods or convenience foods?
- Use mealtime as family time?
- Eat with children at mealtimes so they see you eating and enjoying the same foods?
- Limit snacking before mealtime so children come to the table ready to eat?
- Offer children different kinds of foods so they learn to enjoy a variety of foods?
- Compliment children on good eating habits?
- Celebrate special occasions with a child's favorite meal?
- Serve favorite healthy foods often?
- Know how to read nutritional labels and do so?
- Help children understand nutritional labels so they can, for example, find the fat content on a bag of cookies?

Messages About Nutrition in the School

Schools send messages about healthy foods and eating habits in two general ways. One way is more "formal," using written or otherwise established policies and rules as well as curriculum materials and classroom instruction. These comprise the "what we say" category. The informal category includes behavior and practice—what we actually do in the school environment.

What we do, and what children observe about our behavior, is what we model for them and what they may well try to emulate. In the ideal world, our behavior would be in harmony with our words. However, often this is not the case, for a variety of reasons. The sections that follow are designed to be thought provoking and to encourage you to increase your awareness of what is being modeled in the area of nutrition at your school. You'll find ideas for questions to raise as well as suggestions for change.

The school provides foods for children through cafeteria lunches (the school lunch program) and vending machines. What we serve in the cafeteria and what we offer for sale in vending machines as meals and snacks are revealing. What messages are we communicating to children and youth about what's appropriate and healthy to eat?

The School Cafeteria

School lunches teach children about food choices every day. It is important to look at what we are serving children for lunch to ensure that we are sending the messages we really want to send. We especially need to spot the areas where what we practice is not in keeping with what we teach.

A recent panel pointed out, "Schools should be teaching kids what's best in the classroom—and the cafeteria" (Snider, 1991). Since more than 20 million children eat school lunches each day, the message school cafeterias send is a powerful one. We need to be certain that we are not unwittingly sending children mixed messages about healthy food choices.

What can change? One suggestion made by the U.S. Department of Health and Human Services' *Healthy People 2000* (1991) is that more school lunch programs incorporate the principles of the *Dietary Guide-*

lines for Americans. While these guidelines are used by many schools to develop their meals, their use should be universal.

Healthy People 2000 recommends that we "increase to at least 90 percent the proportion of school lunch and breakfast services that are consistent with the nutritional principles in the *Dietary Guidelines for Americans.*" To meet this objective, school lunches must provide choices that include low-fat foods, vegetables, fruits and whole-grain products. High-fat foods such as french fries and potato chips should appear only infrequently on the menu.

To help children learn to make choices, *Healthy People 2000* also recommends that schools offer "point-of-choice" nutrition information in the school cafeteria. For example, some cafeteria-style restaurants now have an information card by each food listing its nutrient value and calories. Such information would have the added benefit of supporting children's learning experiences in the classroom, allowing them to practice the health knowledge and food selection skills introduced in the classroom.

Educators are role models in the cafeteria as well as in the classroom. When the school staff eat the food prepared at school, they send a positive message about that food. Even if educators fill their plates in the cafeteria and carry the food to a staff lounge, students observe that adults are eating the same food as they are. This action provides a very effective way to model food choices for students.

Salad Bars

Salad bars are becoming increasingly popular in school cafeterias, for a variety of reasons. Children like the texture and colors of salads and the ability to make choices about what they want to eat. Salad bars let students become active participants in the lunch process as they serve themselves and make decisions about what items to choose.

The use of salad bars can increase school lunch participation and, if properly managed, can be less expensive and labor intensive than conventional lunches. One Michigan school district saw such a dramatic increase in participation in school lunches after introducing salad bars that the revenues from the program increased by $50,000 in the first year.

The items used in the salad bar will vary based on seasonal availability. Some items—cheese, cottage cheese, bacon bits and dressings—are often high in fat, but by switching to low-fat versions, including bacon bits, the fat content can be dramatically reduced. Self-service equipment used for salad bars can also become a center for potato and taco bars.

Salad Bar Items with Kid Appeal

- turkey ham
- nonfat cottage cheese
- raisins
- low-fat cheeses
- tomatoes
- cucumbers
- cauliflower
- broccoli
- sunflower seeds
- carrot sticks
- celery sticks
- peppers (green, yellow or red)
- eggs
- mushrooms
- croutons
- chow-mein noodles
- low-fat yogurt
- pudding
- low-fat bacon bits
- alfalfa sprouts
- a variety of low-fat salad dressings
- tofu

Presentation of foods is also important. Adding a cherry to pear halves or serving sliced instead of shredded carrots adds variety without adding food cost. Finger foods are easy and fun to eat, too. Inclusion of other "fun" foods such as pizzas and tacos along with a pleasant and sociable environment can further increase school lunch enjoyment and participation.

Schools have an opportunity to introduce good nutritional habits through the school lunch program. You may not think about the school lunch program as you focus on individual classrooms or curriculum areas, yet the program provides the opportunity to expose students to new or healthy foods and the chance to model healthy food habits during the lunch hours. School staff can also help students develop a love of salads, fresh fruits and other healthy foods—as well as ensure that students get good nutrition and can return to the classroom ready to learn.

Vending Machines

Vending machines have also become a lucrative means for schools to raise funds. Many schools have increased the use of vending machines because of the lack of cafeteria equipment space and the high cost of cafeteria equipment and staffing. The vending machine industry provides attractive and appealing products for all ages.

Technology now allows the dispensing of full meals and allows schools to offer fewer hot lunches or snacks. Even if the number of students using the school lunch program declines, the school still can earn a profit with these machines. This profit makes vending machines even more attractive.

Foods in vending machines often are high in calories and low in nutrients. Vending machines can contain nutritious snacks, but the shelf life of nutritious snacks is not as long as that of processed foods. Ideally, vending machines should be removed from schools, and snacks and lunches should come from the cafeteria.

Self-Assessment: The School Lunch Program

Think about the lunch program at your school. What habits is this program encouraging in students? How can you, as an educator, reinforce and support the nutritional policies of the school food program?

As an educator, do you:

■ Know if students eat well at lunch?

■ Talk to students about the importance of eating a good lunch?

■ Ask students if they enjoyed their lunch?

■ Talk to students about the menu for the week or day so they know what their choices are?

■ Know if your school tells parents what foods the school lunch program offers and what the cafeteria policies are?

■ Know what kinds of foods are served in the cafeteria—processed, fresh, etc.?

■ Eat the foods prepared by your school?

■ Work with the administration or school board to ensure that healthy foods are served?

■ Work with the administration or school board to start a salad bar with low-fat or nonfat salad dressings available if you don't have one?

■ Know what kind of foods students bring in lunches packed from home?

■ Talk to parents or send them information with healthy lunch suggestions?

■ Invite family members to join the class for lunch so that students can share the lunch experience with their families?

■ Know if vending machines are used for the school lunch program?

■ Work to eliminate vending machines or to ensure that they offer healthy choices?

Family Connection: Considerations for Parents

Parents can influence children's attitudes about school lunches, as well. By asking children about their lunch break—what they ate, how it was, with whom they ate—and offering supportive suggestions or just listening, parents can actively demonstrate an interest in the lunch meal. Showing this interest tells children that lunch is an important part of the day.

Self-Assessment: School Lunch Awareness

As a parent, do you:

- Know what kinds of foods your children's school offers at lunch?
- Know if the school prepares its own food or uses packaged meals?
- Ever eat lunch at school with children?
- Know if your children's teachers eat the food offered at school?
- Discuss the lunch menu with children?
- Know how much of the lunch your child eats every day?
- Know if the school has a salad bar?
- Encourage children to eat from the salad bar?
- Talk to children about their lunches each day?
- Offer children a choice of hot lunch or a lunch packed from home?
- Send healthy lunches to school?
- Avoid high-fat and high-sugar items in packed lunches?
- Send easy-to-eat items in packed lunches?
- Know if the school offers whole or low-fat milk?
- Know if vending machines provide lunches?
- Work to remove vending machines or to ensure that they offer healthy choices?

Accepting Diversity of Body Types

People come in a wide variety of shapes and sizes. This diversity is affected by both biological and cultural factors. For example, obesity tends to run in families. Obese parents may have food and activity habits that foster their obesity, but research also supports a conclusion that genetics plays an important role in body weight.

Adults can encourage children to accept body characteristics that can't be changed by modeling acceptance of their own bodies. Adults can also model making healthy choices to change the characteristics that we can control.

The ideal image of slenderness promoted by the mass media and various business interests sets children up for unrealistic expectations. They come to believe that they can attain a certain body size and shape if they just buy or do the "right" things. This ideal ignores the basic reality of human diversity in size and shape and perpetuates the stigma attached to those who stray from the ideal. It furthers the fear of fat that has become endemic in American society.

This cultural ideal is very different from the ideal in many other societies. In some parts of the world where food is scarce, being fat is considered a sign of wealth and carries great prestige. In some countries, children and young adults may be slim and athletic, but adults are expected to be heavy as a sign of maturity and status.

In many parts of the United States, school populations are likely to be multicultural. This diversity is important to keep in mind in developing guidelines for healthy behavior for children and parents.

Suggestions for health-promoting activities are more likely to be acted upon if they are both culturally appropriate and practical. This is particularly true for activities relating to eating habits and body size, since these reflect beliefs and behaviors that often have great emotional and cultural significance.

Food Habits and Body Image

Educators and parents can do a great deal to help children develop a healthy perspective on weight and body size. How you feel about your own and others' body size helps determine what kind of role model you are for children with respect to body image. For example, if you are constantly dieting, you may inadvertently be promoting fear of fat in children and sending a message that constant dieting is important.

Feelings about body size also are demonstrated when we react to others. Statements such as "Ms. Johnson is really putting on weight" or "He can't do that because he's too fat" suggest to children that it's OK to evaluate people and their abilities based on their body size.

Educators may not recognize that they are uncomfortable with overweight or fat children. They may feel critical of students' parents for not eating better or not leading a more fitness-oriented lifestyle. In the classroom, teachers may not call on such students as often as others or may not offer the same kinds of encouragement that they give to other students.

Self-Assessment: Body Image Issues at School

Consider how you may be modeling attitudes about body size in your own behavior and when you interact with other people. As an educator, do you:

- Feel comfortable with your body size?
- Refuse to feel superior to or prejudiced against others because of their weight?
- Encourage healthy eating without talking about gaining or losing weight?

Watch Out For...

- Letting students know you are on a weight-loss diet.
- Talking about dieting or body size with other staff when students can hear.
- Talking about a student's diet progress or body shape when other students can hear.

- Treating overweight children differently from others (e.g., not choosing them for the lead part in a play or thinking they cannot be a contributing member of a soccer team).

- Reacting with surprise when overweight children do well in class.

Dieting and Weight Control

Americans are on a diet roller coaster. We try one diet after another, lose weight, only to gain it back. Most diets don't change the eating habits that contributed to the extra weight. Mass media regularly promote the "ideal" body—especially the ideal female body, although there is pressure on males as well. In 1990, Americans spent $32 billion on weight control products and services. About 65 million Americans are dieting at any given time.

Television programs seldom include children or adults who are large or overweight. Some of the few adult television stars who are overweight have experienced scathing media critiques of their weight, and others have undergone highly publicized weight-loss campaigns—only to regain the weight. What do these kinds of painful experiences model for children, especially children who are larger than average?

Not only do the mass media promote an ideal body type that for many is unattainable, they also promote unrealistic expectations about people's ability to control body size and shape. Advertisements suggest that everybody can have the ideal body. This suggestion perpetuates an intolerant attitude toward people who are fat. Children come to think that people are fat because they have made wrong decisions and they lack self-control. By the time they are six years old, most children think that being fat is "bad." They associate being fat with being lazy, sloppy, dirty and stupid.

Family Connection: Considerations for Parents

Parents are the primary influence on the body image of young children and can play a major role in shaping positive feelings about body size. As children get older, they become more susceptible to the seductive influence of the mass media. Then it becomes even more important for the adults in children's lives to model acceptance of diversity of body types. One of the most powerful ways to do this is to demonstrate acceptance of your own body size and shape.

Children can sense how we feel about body size. Our beliefs and feelings may color our behavior toward them and model a poor self-image. For example, if we are obsessed with being thin, we may be teaching children to be similarly obsessed. Parents need to become more self-aware as they model beliefs and feelings about body shapes and sizes.

Self-Assessment: Body Image Issues at Home

As a parent, do you:

- Feel comfortable about your own body size?
- Feel good about how your children look?
- Regularly compliment children on how they look no matter what size they are?
- Express acceptance of different body shapes and sizes?
- Talk about different body sizes and physical traits in a positive way?
- Comment on the good eating habits of your family?
- Notice that your children are accepting of the way others look?
- Feel comfortable if your children need to wear glasses or braces?

Watch Out For...

- Making comments such as, "Don't eat that. You'll get fat."
- Talking about people's physical appearance in a negative way.
- Weighing yourself often and worrying at the slightest change.
- Having diet products in the home where children can see them.
- Eating different foods from your family because you are dieting.
- Telling children that they are putting on weight, even if you're teasing.
- Thinking that children are too tall, too short, too fat or too thin.
- Telling children that only people with certain body types can play sports (for example, only tall people can play basketball).

Parents and teachers are potent models when it comes to the acceptance of ourselves and others regardless of body type, weight or other physical characteristics. When children see the acceptance of everyone—and all body types—it helps build their self-esteem and helps them learn this same acceptance and compassion.

Talking about nutrition and fitness with young children does not have to include discussion of body fat and weight loss. The emphasis should be that children need proper foods for growth and fitness to feel better and take care of themselves—not to stay thin or lose weight.

When students tease other children about being fat, they are reflecting beliefs and attitudes that they have learned from adults or other models such as those on television and in the movies. Children hear other adults talk about weight loss and the need to have a better-looking body or they hear discussion about other people's weight. This talk gives children the message that these adults are dissatisfied with their bodies and will only be satisfied when they are thin.

Adults promote fear of fat in children by discussing weight and weight loss in front of them. A thin eight-year-old child who fears she must diet because she is "fat" has been bombarded with the thought that to be thin is to be accepted and admired.

Staff members who meet in the hallway and comment, "You're losing weight. Congratulations!" say to students that losing weight is something to be proud of. In this conversation, the fact that weight is the personal quality that is discussed indicates to children how significant it is.

Adults who feel that they must lose weight should reflect on their approach and its impact on the children around them. Frequent dieting is not a healthy approach to weight control. Constant dieting slows down the body's ability to burn calories, making it more difficult to lose weight on each subsequent diet. As people grow older and less active, weight changes occur. The body's metabolism changes and fewer calories are burned through daily routine.

The key to a life without dieting is to increase activity and change eating habits. Reducing the daily consumption of fats and increasing the consumption of foods high in dietary fiber, such as whole grains, fruits and vegetables, can have an impact on weight as the increased fiber moves food through the body and the decreased fat results in less body fat. Regular exercise burns off fat and helps the body stay healthy.

Educators who teach health education or weight loss classes have the opportunity to introduce valuable information that can change lifestyle patterns. How educators feel about body size and weight loss affects what they model for students.

Self-Assessment: Teaching About Weight Control and Health

In this self-assessment, contemplate how you feel about yourself and how you discuss weight control with your students.

As an educator, do you:

- Feel you present a positive image to your students of a person with a healthy lifestyle?

- Feel good during your work day and show enthusiasm about health when you teach?

- Think your students understand that dieting and weight loss are serious activities that are discouraged for young people?

- Encourage students to exercise regularly?

- Include an exercise program such as walking—led by you—in your classes?

- Include nutrition and weight management, rather than weight control, as part of your curriculum for all students?

- Discuss fast foods or processed foods and explain their nutritional value?

- Talk about alternatives to fast foods?

■ Explain that an occasional fast food meal is fine and that moderation is the key?

■ Include parents by sending home information on how to reduce fat and increase activity?

■ Talk with a parent of each child in the class to discuss home eating patterns and offer encouragement to the parents?

■ Talk about lifestyle choices with your students?

Family Connection: Considerations for Parents

Parents have the ability to teach and model to children healthy patterns of eating and exercise. These patterns, not dieting, should be the route to weight control. We need to examine our own healthy behaviors, how we model these behaviors and how we encourage children to develop their own healthy patterns. Parents must think about the healthy patterns of eating and exercise that they would like their children to possess as adults.

Self-Assessment: Weight Control at Home

As a parent, do you:

• Know and accept that there is a wide range of normal weights for children?

• Know what your children weigh right now?

• Talk with your children's physician when children are not present if you have questions or concerns about their weight?

• Know what kinds of foods children eat when you are not around?

• Talk privately with children about how they can manage their body size?

• Take part in daily exercise with children?

• Eat well and exercise regularly?

• Offer the family a healthy diet?

• Help children learn to listen to their own body signals about hunger?

• Keep healthy snack foods at home, foods that are low in fat and high in vitamins, minerals, protein and complex carbohydrates?

• Avoid comparing children?

• Help children change eating and exercise habits instead of dieting?

• Compliment children on their appearance on a regular basis?

Eating Disorders

Dieting by young people of normal or low body weight can cause a threat to their nutritional status and possibly lead them into eating disorders. Two eating disorders, bulimia and anorexia nervosa, have become increasingly common, especially in girls around the age of puberty. These conditions are extreme examples of the harm that is done by promoting an ideal of thinness and a fear of fat. In recent years, a number of prominent actresses and models—who are the embodiment of this rigid ideal—have publicly acknowledged their long-term struggles with eating disorders.

Bulimia is characterized by binge-eating and then purging. Binges may last from a few minutes to several hours and then are followed by periods of self-induced purging through use of vomiting, laxatives, fasting, diets or vigorous exercise. One study of high school girls found that more than 10 percent used vomiting and nearly 5 percent used laxatives to lose weight.

Anorexia nervosa is self-induced starvation. Young people with this condition view themselves as much fatter than they really are and starve themselves to reduce body size. While those who are bulimic may appear normal in weight, girls who are anorexic are often skeleton-like in appearance. Social pressures contribute to both conditions. Some experts suggest that these conditions are related to a fear of growing up or a rebellion against standards set too high by others.

Parents and teachers must be alert to the signs of these conditions among teens. Modeling behavior that is accepting of all body sizes or weights is critical for the early teenage years. Parents who overemphasize weight, control eating behavior or demand perfection may set a pattern that puts pressure on children and leads them to believe that weight control is a condition for love and acceptance.

Educators and parents who foster an acceptance of all body shapes and sizes and who offer an opportunity to learn and experience healthy eating and fitness can help children avoid these disorders.

Other steps to help children with self-image include:

- Discussing media images of thinness—and the fact that few women or men are that thin.

- Pointing out the increase in fit, rather than thin, models, as well as current trends toward showing more diversity of body types and showing disabled models.

- Encouraging the development of a healthy body instead of a thin body.

Sports Nutrition

Young athletes need good nutrition for optimal physical conditioning and performance. Not only do they burn calories in their daily work-outs, but they also can quickly deplete their bodies' storage of protein and carbohydrates.

In the case of sports nutrition, there is a danger that coaches may assume that parents are providing adequate foods, while parents assume that coaches have discussed appropriate foods with the athletes. The parents of athletes need to know what foods their children need, and the coaches need not only to provide this information, but to know that their athletes are eating appropriately.

In addition to teaching sports nutrition, educators need to model sports nutrition. The foods needed by the athlete should be eaten by the adults, too. Coaches who encourage high-carbohydrate, high-protein diets but who sip colas and munch on candy while students work out give the wrong message.

Coaches who encourage athletes to diet to achieve a certain weight before an event are modeling to these students that such dieting is a good approach. Long after these athletes have left the classroom of this coach, these dieting patterns may remain. As an example, wrestling coaches may demand weight loss in an extremely short period of time, giving students the impression that extreme measures are appropriate. Students who have little fat to lose may wind up using diuretics, laxatives and fasting to reach goals. But children can't afford to have their bodies depleted of nutrients when a coach expects them to do so.

Self-Assessment: Nutrition and Training at School

How do you model the need for appropriate nutrition in training? Consider the following self-assessment questions.

As an educator, do you:

■ Model good eating habits to students?

■ Educate students on how the body works when training?

■ Offer training tips to students so they know how to get in shape and stay in shape?

■ Talk with students about sports nutrition so they understand why their bodies need certain nutrients?

■ Distribute information to students and parents on sports nutrition?

■ Understand carbohydrate loading and know how carbohydrates are used by the body during exercise?

■ Encourage students to eat correctly at all times, not just before an event?

Watch Out For...

■ Encouraging excess vitamin intake.

■ Encouraging excessive weight loss for athletes.

■ Telling players that they can't participate unless they meet a certain weight-loss deadline.

■ Encouraging students to lose water weight with diuretics or excessive exercise.

■ Worrying about your own weight and letting your students know it.

■ Undergoing dramatic steps to lose weight.

Family Connection: Considerations for Parents

Parents are a pivotal part of sports nutrition. They need to understand what kinds of foods their children need both at mealtimes and as snacks before training and at meets. Foods high in carbohydrates, fruits such as bananas and oranges, and performance drinks that help supply the nutrients depleted in a workout are good selections.

Parents and coaching staff can work together to help children learn that good nutrition is important to being fit athletes. Parents who encourage athletes to eat nutritionally balanced meals can help establish lifelong patterns of healthy eating. Using the following self-assessment, parents can evaluate their own knowledge of sports nutrition and how they model or encourage healthy eating habits.

Self-Assessment: Sports Nutrition at Home
As a parent, do you:
- Understand what sports nutrition is?
- Know if your children's coach talks about sports nutrition with students?
- Ask the coach to provide information on sports nutrition?
- Know what kinds of food children need at meals and snacks?
- Plan to meet the nutritional needs of children?
- Provide snacks that offer complex carbohydrates and protein before and after training?
- Ask children to help shop for and prepare food?

Watch Out For...
- Letting a child's coach suggest that the child lose weight.
- Encouraging children to lose weight quickly before a sporting event.

Chapter 4

Exercise and Physical Fitness

PHYSICAL FITNESS THROUGH regular exercise can promote health and prevent disease. Physical fitness refers primarily to the efficiency of the cardiovascular system as it transports oxygen. Increased oxygen levels give us more capacity to work and play without feeling tired. Physical fitness also refers to the strength and flexibility of the muscles.

Regular aerobic exercise can help reduce the risk of coronary heart disease, and regular physical activity can prevent and treat conditions such as diabetes, obesity, depression and stress. Exercise is credited with improving self-esteem, aiding in alcohol and other drug treatment programs and improving brain function and cognitive performance.

Even with the increasing interest in exercise and fitness in recent years—including staggering sales of home exercise equipment—only a small percentage of Americans get enough exercise to achieve clear health benefits. Only about 15 to 20 percent of adults participate in appropriate exercise. In students ages ten to eighteen, about 40 percent engage in year-round physical activities, and 36 percent participate in daily physical education classes in school. By grade twelve, it is estimated that nearly half of students do not have physical education in their weekly schedules.

While low-nutrient-density food and television are part of the problem, so is our national fitness strategy for schools. Fewer than one percent of children can earn the Presidential Fitness Award, a national recognition award based on specific criteria. Fitness tests are outmoded, and educators often grade students by performance rather than by participation, leading students who lag behind to give up.

Only from two to five minutes of a typical physical education class are dedicated to strenuous activity. The remaining time is relegated to instruction, discussion or light exercise, which means that students are not getting the appropriate amount of aerobic exercise. Outside school, television and video games are major time takers that contribute nothing to health.

The potential benefits of daily physical education in a school setting are many. Students can become more physically fit and learn to appreciate the relationship between fitness and health. Students can increase their stamina, energy and coordination. They can socialize with their classmates in a noncompetitive setting outside the classroom, learning about self-discipline and about sportsmanship. They can also gain the knowledge and motivation that will carry them into active lifestyles long beyond their school years.

Fitness in the Schools

Schools have a unique opportunity to instill a love of fitness in children. While physical education teachers and coaches are particularly vital to these beliefs, they do not work alone. The school administration's attitude toward fitness is very important.

A school that offers a walking program for teachers or holds annual family fitness days shows the community that it is committed to fitness. A school that encourages children of all abilities, both male and female, to exercise shows its belief that all children can be involved in fitness.

Likewise, parents can bolster what is taught at school and make sure that fitness is a part of daily lives. Parents who ask about physical education classes, participate in family sports, and are concerned with fitness reinforce what is modeled at school.

Fitness skills begin at very young ages. With continued modeling and instruction by both the family and the school, these skills can become habits that will keep children healthy as they grow older.

Many adults can vividly remember their own physical education classes, where grades were based on how many sit-ups they could do, how fast they could run, or how well their team scored in volleyball. For students who could not keep up, physical education classes were often humiliating. Any notion that exercise could be fun was lost.

Today, many adults hope that those days of discouraging and ineffective physical education classes are gone, but they may not be. Schools may not realize how important a physical education teacher is. This person introduces—and models—exercise and fitness. If the teacher does not do so in a positive fashion, or if the school does not place a high value on this position in times when budgets must be trimmed, then we may create a generation of children and youth who hate exercise.

Fewer than half of all American children get enough exercise for minimal levels of fitness. While there is much media attention focused on professional athletes, many schools are not providing appropriate physical education programs for students, nor are students getting the exercise they need at home. In lean economic times, faced with the need to fit in the required number of academic courses each day, schools may cut back on physical education.

Elementary schools often have physical education only once or twice a week, and middle schools may offer these classes only every other year. Schools may wrongly assume that with the increase in adults' interest in fitness, students' fitness needs are being met at home.

Some schools may take the position that it is not their responsibility to keep children fit.

Many physical education programs rely heavily on team sports, which most people do not carry into adulthood. These highly competitive sports, which pit one child or group of children against another, have questionable health benefits. As adults, we may not regularly take part in volleyball, baseball or basketball games, but we may ski, play tennis, run or walk. Yet many schools find it easier to teach team sports, where all the students are active at the same time, rather than sports such as skiing or tennis where some one-on-one instruction may be needed.

The nonteam forms of exercise are often called *lifetime activities*. Lifetime fitness activities focus on not only the physical skills, but the knowledge, attitudes and cognitive skills that will keep young people physically active far beyond their school days. Schools play an important part in offering skills to develop active lifestyles that will carry over into adulthood. Physical education teachers and the administrations that support them have a responsibility to introduce and model exercise and fitness.

If a school offers physical education only every other year, the school sends a message that this activity is not important. Similarly, if a school promotes only team sports, then students assume that team sports are the only way to exercise. As models, these schools model the premise that exercise is not important or that the only valued modes of exercise are highly competitive team sports.

Students recognize the disparities between what adults teach them at school and how these adults actually conduct themselves in the school environment. Educators who teach physical education are perhaps more vulnerable to these kinds of comparisons between what is said and what is practiced. However, role models cannot work in a vacuum; if messages about health and fitness are to be effective, the larger social environment must also support them. Keep this in mind as you work through the self-assessments in this chapter.

Self-Assessment: Fitness in Your Life

No one expects you alone to take full responsibility for children's exercise habits. But do recognize that as an adult with a high level of authority—and particularly if you are a physical education teacher—you can be an important influence when it comes to students' lifetime fitness choices.

Consider your own attitudes toward fitness and exercise. What is the role of fitness in your life?

As an educator, do you:

- Believe regular exercise is important?
- Exercise regularly?
- Feel good after exercising?
- Exercise when students can see you?
- Encourage students to exercise with you?
- Understand the value of fitness in overall health?
- Regularly participate in lifetime fitness activities?
- Think you will still be exercising regularly ten years from now?

Self-Assessment: Fitness at School

Attitudes promoted by the school are powerful models to children. Schools with strong physical education programs suggest to students—and parents—that fitness is important. In this next assessment, consider the role of your school in fitness and your own role in promoting fitness to students.

As an educator, do you:

- Believe your school promotes fitness?
- Offer daily physical education in your school for all ages?

■ Believe that physical education is important?

■ Know whether physical education classes are structured so that more time is spent on activity than instruction?

■ Know whether your school offers a developmentally appropriate and sequential fitness program?

■ Know whether your school requires physical education teachers to be certified?

■ Receive inservice training if classroom teachers teach physical education?

■ Know whether your physical education program focuses on lifetime skills?

■ Reward students with special events that are active (such as bowling, miniature golf or swimming)?

■ Encourage students to spend recess time outside?

■ Talk about fitness with students?

■ Organize class fitness days?

■ Include the entire school in activities such as a school walking program?

■ Include family members in activities such as a one-day walking event?

Ideas for Classroom Activities to Promote Fitness

Fitness activities do not have to be confined to physical education classes. There are many ways to encourage fitness in the classroom and to integrate fitness into the curriculum.

In Art...

■ Conduct events such as poster competitions to highlight the role of physical fitness.

- Create bumper stickers or other graphics to promote exercise.
- Draw pictures of people engaged in activity.
- Use clay to sculpt body tone and muscles.

In Language Arts...

- Conduct and publish a survey on physical fitness in the school.
- Roleplay with students about interest in exercise.
- Have students write essays or stories on why to exercise.
- Ask students to follow the progress of a particular athlete and report on it.
- Put together a dictionary of terms relating to fitness and exercise.
- Have students write about sports nutrition.

In Math...

- Estimate actual age versus chronological age using health appraisals.
- Estimate the number of calories burned in different exercises.
- Calculate the number of grams of fat in a typical school lunch and estimate how much exercise it would take to burn them off.
- Calculate heart rate, target heart rate and recovery heart rate based on age and fitness levels.

In Science...

- Take part in health-risk appraisals, using a computer.
- Study the effects of exercise on body chemistry, stress, endorphins, etc.
- Discuss nutrition and how it affects body chemistry.
- Talk about the theory and practice of sports nutrition.

The Role of the Physical Education Teacher

The physical education teacher has a special part to play in the modeling of fitness to students. This teacher's role is to actively participate in fitness, to talk about fitness and to encourage students to experience a variety of physical activities.

Educators need to motivate children to develop lifelong habits. Educators continue to search for avenues to increase exercise among students and their families. Families are important because there is a direct link between adult exercise habits and children's impressions of fitness. Physical education programs that are fun let students know that exercise does not have to be boring or painful.

Educators have an opportunity to instill in students a sense of satisfaction that comes from learning and improving physical skills. With these skills comes the added benefit that health can be enhanced through exercise. This encouragement is especially important among young children who do not routinely seek exercise in their own lives. Older children must care enough about themselves, and have high enough self-esteem, to want to exercise. School fitness programs that let students know what they can do and promote an interest in exercise can have a long-lasting influence.

That educators can influence lifelong habits is not a new thought. An English teacher with a love of literature may instill an interest in reading that lasts a lifetime. A science teacher who takes the children out into the woods for a lesson in field biology excites their interest. The same can be true of a physical education teacher.

An educational environment that promotes an active lifestyle can help develop students who are enthusiastic about exercise, both within and outside the school. Talking about—and illustrating—improvements in cardiovascular rates clearly demonstrates the health benefits of exercise.

Self-esteem, too, can be positively influenced by exercise. Just being fit can improve self-esteem. So can fitness programs designed around achieving individual goals instead of group activities. A noncompetitive environment is a pivotal factor in increasing self-esteem. Group activities should not revolve around a score. Students can take turns being referee, which also increases their knowledge of the rules.

Self-Assessment: Modeling Fitness Habits at School

Early development of positive attitudes toward exercise can play an important part in guiding students to an active lifestyle. The physical education teacher is a significant model for students and can help instill lifelong fitness habits.

The self-assessment that follows is designed especially for the physical education teacher, although the questions are also useful for other educators. Students who have fun and learn fitness skills in physical education classes will carry that enthusiasm into the rest of the day.

As you read through the questions, think about the role the physical education teacher plays in modeling a lifetime of fitness habits. The questions encourage you to consider beliefs as well as actions.

As a physical education teacher, do you:

- Believe that fitness is important in daily life and convey this to students?

- Exercise regularly?

- Wear exercise clothing for class?

- Take part in activities with your students?

- Think your students see you as actively helping them reach fitness goals?

- Use a physical activity log to help students keep personal records of their exercise?

■ Design individual fitness goals that students can attain?

■ Conduct a systematic and periodic assessment of the physical fitness of children to know how students are progressing?

■ Recognize students for participating in fitness testing and for their progress?

■ Give parents general information on fitness and report on their children's fitness status?

■ Inform parents of the structure of your physical education program?

■ Think parents know what takes place in your physical education classes?

■ Use a buddy system when working out to encourage student participation?

■ Compliment individual students on fitness and appearance as a result of exercise?

■ Concentrate on lifetime fitness activities?

■ Talk about the role of the family in fitness?

■ Use a variety of enjoyable activities in your curriculum?

■ Know if your students are having fun in and look forward to your class?

Self-Assessment: Promoting Student Fitness

The types of exercises and fitness activities you introduce in physical education classes are also important. These activities need to be fun to do and contribute to fitness, but they also need to offer instruction and entice students to continue them outside the classroom. Here, ask yourself about the kinds of exercises that students are exposed to in school and the level of fitness they reach from these activities. These questions may inspire you to put some of these ideas into practice.

As a physical education teacher, do you:

■ Evaluate cardiovascular benefits of physical activities before choosing exercises to teach?

■ Focus on activities with cardiovascular benefits?

■ Consider the other benefits of activities (e.g., developing muscular flexibility, strength and endurance; enhancing coordination, agility and balance; improving reaction time) in making exercise choices?

■ Use both aerobic and anaerobic exercises in your program?

■ Talk to students about the benefits of different kinds of exercise?

■ Use stretching, warm-up and cool-down exercises?

■ Offer actual instruction in a sport, along with daily participation?

■ Talk about the types of clothing used in different sports?

■ Include sports nutrition in your teaching?

■ Discourage weight gain or weight loss for competition purposes?

■ Discuss common fitness training injuries and precautions to take?

■ Develop enrichment programs for before or after school or during lunch time?

■ Develop and advise clubs, teams or other groups for specific activities (such as swimming or biking)?

■ Promote physical fitness through special events such as fun runs, bicycle rodeos, physical fitness days, triathlons?

■ Work with other teachers to promote fitness?

■ Identify and mark trails for walking or jogging on school property?

■ Promote after-school aerobic exercise classes for faculty and staff?

■ Provide students with a directory on community recreation and fitness activities?

■ Work with your school administration to promote a cohesive fitness program?

Family Connection: Considerations for Parents

Parents are important models of fitness. The home environment can inspire children to include fitness in their daily lives. Parents' fitness habits and attitudes are what children see on a daily basis. Does the family do activities together, such as skiing, biking or walking? Do children sense that fitness is a family activity that everyone enjoys?

Many parents may not have a good understanding of the physical education (PE) programs at school. Parents are pivotal in the physical education process, as it is their commitment to overall fitness and their support of the school's efforts that tell children that fitness is indeed essential.

The following self-assessment can help parents examine family attitudes toward fitness and empower them to find out more about the school's PE program.

Self-Assessment: Fitness at Home

Family Fitness

As a parent, do you:

- Promote fitness and exercise at home?
- Exercise regularly?
- Take part in lifetime fitness activities such as walking, swimming, biking or tennis?
- Make time for family activities such as walking, biking, swimming or skiing?
- Let children see you as an active person?
- Think your children will grow up to be active if they follow in your footsteps?
- Wear the right clothing for your fitness activities?

Watch Out For...

- Having fitness equipment you don't use.
- Saying, "I'll start exercising tomorrow."

(continued)

School Fitness

As a parent, do you:

- Understand the PE program in your children's school?
- Know how often students have PE?
- Know if all grade levels have PE?
- Know how children are graded in PE?
- Talk to the PE teacher during parent/teacher conferences?
- Get information on fitness from the school?
- Know if children's teachers take part in PE classes or watch from the sidelines?
- Talk with children about PE classes?
- Make sure children have the exercise clothing or shoes they need?
- Know if fitness testing is used in the school?
- Understand that PE is important to children's lives?
- See educators actively involved in fitness activities such as running or walking?
- Help children take part in after-school sports?
- Help children stay physically fit?
- Get involved with children's sports (for example, attend events or parent meetings, offer to coach or to help the coach)?

Avoiding Stereotypes in Physical Education

Teachers of all subjects and all grade levels need to be aware of children's differences and teach their students to accept—and appreciate—these differences. There are many types of differences, from those that are related to cultural or ethnic background, to those perceived to be related to gender, to more idiosyncratic conditions or situations unique to each child.

In teaching physical education, there is a special need for sensitivity to certain stereotypes or biases. For example, both teachers and students may have ideas about gender that can lead to unfair exclusion of children from activities.

The activities of boys' and girls' physical education classes may vary greatly. Boys may play basketball or football. Girls may play volleyball or run. Girls may not be encouraged to be athletic. Organized sports for girls may be nonexistent—despite laws requiring that girls have the same opportunities as boys.

Physical education classes can be especially painful for children who are overweight. They may be unable to keep up with the class during an activity and may experience ridicule or social isolation. In a math or science class, these students can be equals. But when playing basketball or running laps, they are at a disadvantage.

Physical education teachers are in a unique position to offer support to children in maintaining their weight or achieving weight loss. If teachers are skilled in assessing body composition and administering fitness tests, they can help students achieve their weight and fitness goals.

Educators have a responsibility to teach and model tolerance, compassion and fairness, allowing students the opportunity to do their best with what they have. To do so, educators must be aware of their own attitudes and beliefs as well as those of the students.

Lifetime fitness activities are much more likely than competitive sports to be appropriate for all students. These activities allow students with varying abilities to set individual goals, see progress and feel good in the process.

Coaches have the task of teaching a skill and encouraging and developing that skill. Coaches have a similar responsibility to be even-handed in instruction. Trying out for a team sport is an intense experience, and being cut may mean that children will never again decide to put themselves on the line for a sport. Physical education teachers and coaches can develop budding athletes and instill a life-long love of fitness. They can also turn off students so that they will never want to do any more than the minimum required in the physical education class.

Self-Assessment: Fitness Strategies at School

Approaches to physical fitness in physical education classes are the topic of this self-assessment. Will students leave school with healthy attitudes toward fitness? Is there stereotyping within the physical education program? Are all students equally challenged and included in fitness goals?

As a physical education teacher or coach, do you:

■ Realize your role in building self-esteem?

■ Know if physical education classes for boys and girls are similar in your school?

■ Encourage girls to be active in athletics?

■ Know if extracurricular sports such as soccer and baseball include both boys and girls?

■ Teach both boys and girls?

■ Offer encouragement to all students, regardless of weight or athletic ability, to achieve their goals?

■ Make sure classmates do not tease children about their weight?

■ Offer activities that all students can do?

■ Encourage all students, regardless of weight or athletic ability, to take part in extracurricular activities?

■ Regularly talk to each student's parents just as other teachers do?

■ Encourage students to try different types of sports to find a satisfying activity?

■ Make team cuts with sensitivity?

Watch Out For...

■ Making comments suggesting that girls or boys can't do certain activities.

- Treating students differently due to gender, weight or athletic ability.
- Allowing students to denigrate others.

Chapter 5

Substance Use Prevention

ADULTS CAN BEGIN TO teach many health behaviors when children are very young. Healthy behaviors such as washing hands and brushing teeth are easily modeled on a daily basis, and their benefits are simple to explain. Teaching children the benefits of a substance-free lifestyle is more difficult.

For one thing, preventing substance use means teaching children about behaviors to avoid and actions not to take. This teaching is more confusing for children than promoting positive actions that they can take to stay healthy. It can be more confusing for adults, too. Adults may have a hard time explaining to children why they should avoid smoking, drinking or using drugs. After all, in American society, these substances are pervasive, and their use seems socially acceptable.

The lure of substance use may be great. Children can experience a good deal of social pressure to use various substances. And they may well see adult behavior that directly contradicts the adults' spoken message. Because substances such as nicotine and alcohol are addictive, the adults in a child's life may not be able to control their own behavior. As a result, children get mixed messages about the use of these substances.

High self-esteem may enhance children's ability to stand up to peer pressure to use these substances. Therefore, helping children to develop high self-esteem is an important component of any substance use prevention effort.

In an ideal world, the messages children get from their social milieu would be consistent with the educational content they learn and the behavior of adults they admire and emulate. While we live in an imperfect world, we can try to increase our awareness of our social environment and our own behavior as it affects those around us. Then we can begin to work toward making positive changes.

Tobacco Use

What do children learn about tobacco use from the social environment? They learn that American society, by and large, condones smoking. Smoking sections are allowed in restaurants, airports, stores, bowling alleys, malls, parks, buses and many other public places where children spend time. Cigarettes are widely available in vending machines and at the check-out counters of convenience and grocery stores.

This situation is changing in some states and cities, however. In California, for example, many cities are putting strict "no smoking" laws in place. In San Luis Obispo, California, smoking is not allowed in any public place, including all bars and restaurants. However, many of children's role models may smoke. Twenty-nine percent of all school personnel smoke, for example.

Media Images

Advertising is one of the most prominent sources of the message that smoking is acceptable. Tobacco companies spend millions of dollars on advertising each year, and the people in these ads appear glamorous and exciting. In print and on billboards, advertisements portray smokers as beautiful, athletic, prosperous, happy—and healthy. Children see the people in these ads and imagine their own futures as successful and attractive adults.

Young children also are attuned to other characters appearing in cigarette ads. A cartoon character appearing in a cigarette advertisement is widely identifiable by children and adults. Studies indicate that the use of the cartoon character may have helped the company increase sales in the youth (under-18) market.

Although tobacco advertising is now prohibited on television, children still see smokers in television programs and in movies. Thus, children may perceive smoking as a "grown-up" or "cool" thing to do. Very young children often use pencils, straws or candy cigarettes to imitate cigarette smoking.

Pervasive film and television portrayals of cigarette smoking contribute to the fact that young people consistently and substantially overestimate the prevalence of smoking among adults. Smoking appears to youth to be a low-risk activity and a symbol of adult behavior. Perhaps because of this perception, youth are more likely to experiment with and become dependent on cigarettes. More than 90 percent of all smokers began smoking before age 18.

Fortunately, few network television programs now feature characters who smoke. Advocates for health and against smoking have appealed to the industry to closely monitor the number of characters in movies who use tobacco. Over time, as smoking becomes less acceptable, perhaps such characters will be phased out.

Counteracting the Advertisements

The rules children live by primarily come from parents and teachers. Yet certain media images do not support the rules. Children may well wonder which group is telling the truth—parents and teachers or advertisers?

If we discover that we are inadvertently promoting an unhealthy action to children, we have it in our power to change our behavior. For example, if we discover that we are not washing our hands before meals even though we ask children to do so, we can alter our behavior by washing our hands. With advertising, we are powerless to change the message.

From an early age, children must be educated about tobacco use and advertising. They can begin to understand that businesses are trying to sell a product and get us to use tobacco so that they can make a profit. It may be difficult to explain why this advertising is allowed and why our government lets cigarette smoking be promoted. Young children think that the president or some other "good person" should stop these ads.

Children can be taught that tobacco is big business. Tobacco companies have a vested interest in limiting the information that the public receives on the hazards of tobacco use. Magazines need advertising to make money. Some people believe that powerful advertisers such as tobacco companies can even influence the content of magazines they advertise in. For example, magazines that carry more advertisements for cigarettes seem less likely to carry articles on the dangers of smoking.

The School Environment

One way that schools can do their part to help create consistency in the messages children get about substance use is to adopt a drug-free school policy. The policy should include tobacco as well as alcohol and other drugs and should extend to cover extracurricular events and meetings held on campus.

Schools should be particularly clear about their nonsmoking policy. Allowing smoking in a teacher's lounge indicates to students that smoking is fine as long as it is in a special place. Students who pass the lounge door will smell the smoke. Anyone leaving a smoking lounge—even a nonsmoker—carries the scent of tobacco for hours. Educators who tell students not to smoke and then return to the classroom with smoke on their breath or clothing give students the message that adults can smoke and that the nonsmoking "rule" applies only to children.

Student opinion surveys show that young people overestimate the number of teachers who smoke. Perhaps the social environments of most schools make it appear that more adults smoke than is actually the case. Having designated areas where staff smoke may contribute to this perception.

Adults should take every possible step to keep children in a smoke-free environment. We should clearly tell those around us that smoking is not acceptable.

Self-Assessment: Messages About Tobacco Use

Consider the hidden messages that children receive about the use of cigarettes. Do you provide any of these hidden messages? What positive modeling messages can you give?

As an educator, do you:

- Avoid smoking cigarettes?

- Know the health effects of smoking and of breathing second-hand smoke?

- Attempt to keep a smoke-free environment at home?

- Support a smoke-free environment at school?

■ Seek to make the school a smoke-free campus?

■ Take part in the American Cancer Society's national smoke-out day activities with your classroom?

■ Encourage other staff to quit smoking and offer support when they do?

■ Urge the school to offer smoking cessation classes in its employee assistance program?

■ Educate students about tobacco advertising?

■ Educate students about the health risks of tobacco use?

■ Ask your class to write to tobacco companies about their advertising?

If you smoke, do you:

■ Avoid smoking on or off campus during the school day?

■ Avoid smoking in public areas where children may see you?

Watch Out For...

■ Carrying cigarettes around with you at school.

■ Smoking in your car and then using it to transport students.

■ Sending mixed messages about smoking to students.

Smoking in Public Places

Many businesses now have no-smoking policies to keep work and public environments smoke free. However, employees may smoke outside the entrance, and visitors may see a group of cigarette users as they enter. The building is smoke free, but the message still is conveyed to children that smoking is OK in certain locations.

Family Connection: Considerations for Parents

Environmental tobacco smoke is responsible for higher rates of respiratory infections and other immune system problems. Many nonsmokers in the United States are worried about the health consequences of secondhand smoke.

It is estimated that nearly half the children in the United States live in households where someone smokes. Children with asthma or other chronic respiratory problems are particularly at risk when they live in households with environmental tobacco smoke.

Striving to maintain a smoke-free environment illustrates to children our commitment to keeping them healthy and free from smoke. This may mean that we smoke outside or that we smoke only in designated areas that are well-ventilated. This commitment also means we must ask the same of visitors who smoke.

When visiting other homes where smokers reside, we should ask the smokers to avoid smoking in the presence of children. No-smoking rules should also be adopted for events involving children, such as birthday parties or scout meetings.

It is helpful for parents to reflect on the messages they send their children about tobacco use. Do children see their parents actively working to keep cigarette smoke out of their lives? If children grow up adopting their parents' habits and attitudes toward smoking, will they be smokers or nonsmokers?

Self-Assessment: Messages About Smoking at Home

As a parent, do you:
- Keep your home smoke free?
- Keep parts of your home (such as children's bedrooms) smoke free?
- Ask guests to smoke outside?
- Ask others not to smoke around your family?
- Ask to be seated in nonsmoking sections in restaurants?
- Talk about tobacco advertising with your children?
- Know if your children's school has a smoke-free policy?
- Work toward a smoke-free school?
- Know if your school teaches children about the dangers of tobacco use?
- Offer to help at school when children are learning about preventing the use of tobacco?

(continued)

- Encourage friends or family to quit smoking?
- Know if parents of your children's friends smoke when your child visits?
- Tell children about health problems related to smoking?

Watch Out For...
- Keeping cigarettes where children can see them.
- Buying cigarettes in front of children.
- Offering cigarettes to others.
- Smoking in front of children.
- Sending children to buy cigarettes.

Understandably, smokers may resent being sent to undesirable locations to smoke. Compromises can be struck by allowing smokers to use areas that are less public.

Most restaurants now give customers a choice of eating in a smoking or nonsmoking section. Choosing the nonsmoking sections lets children know that we appreciate the choice and that we choose to stay away from smoke. Telling the restaurant "It doesn't matter which section we dine in" says to children, "It's fine for us to sit in the cigarette smoke." It is not fine to sit in cigarette smoke; secondhand smoke is a health hazard.

Children need to understand that staying away from smoke is the right choice to make. Caregivers have a responsibility to keep children away from smoke, thereby providing the message that we are concerned about the health of those in our care.

Suggestions for Smokers

In an ideal world, no one would smoke. But people do smoke, and many smokers are unable or unwilling to quit. It may be more difficult to raise nonsmokers in a smoking environment, but it can be done.

Adults must be truthful and tell children that smoking is an addiction and that quitting is very difficult. Adults who smoke should clearly explain that smoking is a personal choice and although it may not be a good one, it is one the adult made. The teacher or parent may say, "I don't know why I started smoking, but I did. Now I cannot quit. I know it is not good for me to smoke. I hope that you make better choices than I did."

It also is helpful for children to see smokers trying to break the habit. Not only do they see the commitment of the smoker to ending this practice, but they begin to understand the true addiction of nicotine as the smoker works through the process of quitting.

What can schools do to help smokers? First, schools need to clearly explain that smoking is not permitted on school property. The administration may need to explain that this is not a punishment but that because modeling of smoking does take place, this rule is in the best interests of the children.

Next, schools should have in place an employee assistance program (EAP) that can help smokers if they want help. If such a program doesn't exist, schools should find a local health care organization that sponsors smoking cessation classes and refer educators to that program. Helping educators pay for the class can show the school's commitment.

Parents who smoke need to be equally honest with their children. If they wish to quit smoking, perhaps their employer's EAP can help. Smoking cessation programs are also available in most communities through organizations such as the American Lung Association or the American Cancer Society.

Smoking is not a habit that we want our children to possess. With care in how we model smoking and clear answers to questions about smoking, children can begin to see how much better off they are if they never start to smoke.

Alcohol and Other Drugs

Drug use is a serious problem among teenagers today. It is also a problem for many adults, including the adults children respect and admire. For example, one in ten school staff members is addicted to alcohol. Alcohol is associated with half of all homicides, suicides and deaths from motor vehicle crashes.

Like smoking, social drinking of alcohol is widely considered acceptable in our society. Happy hours and "TGIF" events exemplify institutionalized drinking, where drinking is the primary activity.

Many celebrations include alcohol. Holiday dinners often include wine or cocktails; family gatherings may include a keg of beer; and the birth of a new baby may be celebrated with a bottle of champagne. Drinking alcohol is seen as a way to make occasions festive.

Advertising and the media play an enormous role in the modeling of alcohol and other drug use. Prime-time television programs feature bars as part of everyday life, where people gather to discuss their work day. Movies depict social drinking and other drug use. In many movies, even the "good guys" use drugs but somehow appear to have it under control.

During the holiday season, advertisements portray the warmth and happiness of this time of year—along with a particular beer or liquor. Beer commercials often captivate children with their cleverness or humor. This approach to alcohol leads children to believe that drinking is pleasurable.

Advertisements about alcohol, like those for cigarettes, provide harmful models for children. We must encourage children to think critically about advertising. We can also help them think about characters in movies or on television who are portrayed as regular drinkers by raising the issue and asking them if drinking is a healthy and safe thing to do. We can let them know that we do not think that it is.

A more forthright step is to write to television programs that show the social acceptability of alcohol or other drugs. An entire class could write letters to a television network if a character on one of their favorite shows uses these substances.

The mass media provide powerful models, and their role in children's lives makes positive modeling by teachers and parents even more important.

Self-Assessment: Educators and Alcohol

Educators may think they are exempt from questions about alcohol use because they see children only during school hours. Yet some educators may drink alcohol at lunch or after work in a setting where students can observe them. Students may detect alcohol on the breath even if mints or gum are used to mask it.

Educators are one of the most effective tools in battling students' use of alcohol and other drugs. Educators have the responsibility to teach by what they do as well as by what they say. Leading by example is a perfect way to motivate students.

Many schools offer curriculum materials on drug use prevention. But the impact of these programs is negated if educators model unhealthy use of the substances. Reflect on your own attitudes and behaviors concerning alcohol. To deliver messages about substance use prevention, we need to be credible with students.

As an educator, do you:

■ Avoid drinking alcohol at lunch on school days?

■ Avoid drinking alcohol with other teachers after school or at school parties?

■ Avoid drinking alcohol to the point of intoxication?

■ Avoid talking about "partying" when you're with students?

- Avoid drinking alcohol in public settings (such as family restaurants) where students may see you?

- Always appoint a designated driver if you are drinking alcohol?

Drugs: Licit and Illicit

Nearly all the questions we've raised about alcohol can also be raised about other drugs. And, with some drugs, there are important legal issues and ramifications. If an educator has a drug-use problem, other educators should watch for modeling of unhealthy behaviors to students and urge the educator with a problem to get help. Employee assistance programs are widely available; they may be able to help educators who are motivated to change their behavior.

Educators and parents should be aware that drug modeling may also occur in the use of prescription or over-the-counter drugs. A teacher who has a cold may take an over-the-counter remedy in front of children during the school day. If a headache strikes in midday, a teacher may swallow aspirin without thinking that students might not know what kind of pills he's taking.

Parents may purchase over-the-counter drugs in front of children without explanation. A parent comes down with a suspected case of strep throat and digs into the medicine cabinet for three-year-old antibiotics. A physician prescribes an antibiotic, but the parent feels better and stops taking the medication before the bottle is empty.

In these situations, children receive hidden messages about drugs from parents and educators. They see adults taking pills and assume that taking drugs is fine.

Young children should be taught to take medicine only from a parent or a trusted caregiver. Educators who are asked to give medication at school should find a quiet place to administer the drugs so that other students do not watch. (They should also be aware of all local and state laws related to administering drugs to students.)

Although a teacher, a trusted person, is providing the medication in

Family Connection: Considerations for Parents

If children are to understand that alcohol and other drugs are potential hazards to their health, adults must not only speak clearly on this subject, but they must act clearly as well. We may be giving children confusing messages if we tell them to avoid these substances but we use them ourselves. The following self-assessment focuses on alcohol, a legal drug in common use.

The role of the parent and the home environment is pivotal in forming beliefs about drinking and drug use. Children who grow up with little exposure to alcohol are less likely to have problems with substance use. Problem drinking, for example, is more common in families with vague and inconsistent drinking practices, where one parent favors drinking and the other is opposed, and where standards for drinking are different for men than for women.

In examining the modeling that they provide concerning alcohol, parents must contemplate their own habits and attitudes on this subject. Do children often see alcohol in the home? Do they observe adults who are intoxicated? What do they think when parents offer guests a drink? Do the attitudes parents convey support what they want for their children?

Self-Assessment: Messages About Alcohol at Home

As a parent, do you:
- Make it clear that use of too much alcohol is not acceptable?
- Avoid pressuring people to drink alcohol?
- Make it clear that drinking too much is not funny?
- Offer guests non-alcoholic drinks as well as alcoholic drinks?
- Never let guests drive home after drinking?

Watch Out For...
- Drinking alcohol as a way to escape problems.
- Drinking alcohol or using other drugs after work because you had a bad day.
- Drinking to intoxication.
- Allowing children to observe intoxicated adults.
- Leaving liquor bottles out for children to see or obtain.
- Always including alcohol in family events, parties or celebrations.
- Rewarding children with an alcoholic drink for a special occasion.
- Buying alcohol when children are present.

this case, other students looking on would not know why their classmate is taking a drug. Students might see the special attention this child gets from the teacher when taking the medication and believe that good feelings are associated with taking some kind of drug.

Prescription or over-the-counter medications should not be left out in the open. Not only might a small child take the medication, but its presence suggests that pill use by anyone at any time is acceptable.

Medication is, of course, useful and important under many circumstances. Adults must be observant and aware of their role as models for children when they use these substances.

Modeling a Drug-Free Lifestyle

Children need healthy modeling concerning the use of alcohol and other drugs. In addition to avoiding negative modeling, adults can support the position that use of these substances is potentially hazardous. Adolescents are likely to find themselves in social settings where alcohol or drugs are present. The higher their self-esteem and the more positive models they have in their lives, the more likely they are to be able to withstand peer pressure and make healthy choices.

Self-Assessment: Modeling a Healthy Lifestyle

Consider the positive modeling you provide for children. What kinds of activities do you promote that build self-esteem? Are you active and happy? Do you model these attributes? Do you show that being happy does not require use of alcohol or other drugs?

As an educator, do you:

- ■ Talk with students about alcohol and other drugs and explain their harmful effects?

- ■ Communicate a clear statement of your feelings about alcohol and other drug use?

- ■ Take advantage of "teachable moments" when students are asking questions and ready to learn?

- ■ Take a personal inventory of your tobacco, alcohol and other drug use habits and their impact on students?

- ■ Have a strong sense of self and feel comfortable with your identity and values?

- ■ Encourage healthy, creative, substance-free activities at school?

- ■ Involve students in planning activities and programs that reinforce a drug-prevention message?

- ■ Participate in and promote fitness activities, showing that you value a healthy body?

- ■ Look for ways to weave prevention information into your curriculum?

- ■ Offer a substance-use-prevention (and self-esteem-building) curriculum in the classroom?

- ■ Take every opportunity to build self-esteem among students so that when they are approached with opportunities for substance use they have the skills to say no?

- ■ Talk about decision-making and communication skills in your classroom?

- ■ Create an atmosphere of trust in the classroom and encourage students to talk about their problems or fears?

- ■ Take the time to talk about alcohol or tobacco advertising and how advertising can shape children's beliefs?

- ■ Encourage the development of strong school anti-drug policies?

- ■ Communicate openly with parents to create a sense of community?

Chapter 6

Stress Management: Personal and Social Skills for Success

SIMPLY PUT, STRESS IS the feeling of being under pressure. This pressure affects children and adults in many different ways. Stress may be caused by a job change, a new baby or a divorce.

But it is not just major life events that trigger stress. Research now shows that even daily stressors can be hard to handle for some people. Daily hassles such as oversleeping, bouncing a check or forgetting to put out the garbage can add up.

Stress affects people in different ways. One person is extremely agitated at missing a train while another uses the time to read the paper—and enjoys it. The possibility of losing a job immobilizes one worker while her colleague looks forward to a new opportunity. Stress can cause pain and discouragement or inspire determination and motivation.

Stress operates in the school setting in hundreds of ways. Educators who are easily frazzled by daily dilemmas may be short tempered with their students. An administrator going through a divorce may place unrealistic demands on the staff. Even the stress of a common cold can tire out a teacher, and this change can leave students jumpy and irritable.

Students also experience stress at home. Mom may be starting a new job. Dad might be an alcoholic. A sibling may have a drug problem. Grandpa may move in because he can't live on his own. An exchange student may be an exciting visitor but bring great changes to a household. Students may walk in the school door having already experienced a stressful morning. Mom left home early for a meeting. Dad forgot to pack lunch or give the student lunch money.

After a start like this, students may have a difficult time settling into the classroom routine. Most parents have discovered through experience that an outburst with children in the morning—such as yelling at them to hurry up or a battle over eating breakfast—can turn the entire day into a disaster. Children may not recover from the stress of the morning in time to function at an attentive and participatory level in school.

Children today must learn to cope with many different kinds of pressure. Those who do so are better students, have fewer problems as they reach adolescence and grow up to be adults who are happier, healthier and better able to handle the stresses in their lives.

Several studies show that lifelong patterns for coping with stress are learned in childhood. The resilient child, who can deal with many different types of stress, often learns these coping techniques at a very young age. The ways children learn to cope with the stresses of childhood are carried into adulthood.

Children take their cues from adults on how to handle stress. A parent going berserk when the milk is left on the counter suggests to children that more serious problems, such as a bad grade or a lost backpack, could send the parent into orbit. An educator who is late for school and then gets angry at her students for not performing well on a test sends the message that minor hassles mean we should get upset and angry and that poor performance means punishment. To minimize the stress in children's lives, we as adults must function effectively, seek solutions to our own problems, resolve conflicts and manage our own stress.

The Effects of Stress on the Body

Stress can have a significant impact on the body, and many people who are under stress notice certain body signals. When your body is exposed to stress, many things happen. The digestive system shuts down, and you may lose your appetite or notice "butterflies" in your stomach. Heart rate, blood pressure, breathing rate, blood flow to muscles, blood sugar and perspiration all increase. Blood flow to the extremities decreases, causing cold or numb sensations in the fingers and toes. Certain nutrients in the body are quickly utilized during stress. Vitamin C, for example, is immediately used by the body and, within minutes, a day's supply might be gone.

Many activators, or stressors, can trigger these reactions. Lack of sleep or exercise, inadequate diet, illness, injury, smoking, alcohol or other drug use can stress the body. Social situations can be stressful as well. Young students may be upset if another child is taunting or critical. Children who have few friends or a poor support system at home may find it difficult to deal with daily pressures.

Students with low self-esteem may be easily rattled by a teacher's questioning of a homework assignment. An embarrassing or frustrating situation may be laughable for one student but catastrophic for another. Educators who are extremely demanding or unclear, school settings that are overwhelming or confusing, poor grades, even the thought of an upcoming test can be more than some children can handle.

As adults, we can often sense when we are under stress. We may develop headaches or an upset stomach. Consequently, we may choose to spend a couple of hours in a hammock with a book, go for a long bike ride or take a nap.

Children usually are not sophisticated enough to know that the headache or upset stomach comes from stress. Their behavior changes and they do not know why. Parents and educators may also see changes but not recognize the cause. Stress symptoms are really the body's way of telling us that we are experiencing some kind of difficulty.

Stress Signals

Many of the following stress signals appear when the body is under stress. Think about what is going on in your life if, for example, you suddenly stop sleeping at night and have headaches or stomachaches all day long. Other symptoms of too much stress include:

- crying easily and for no reason
- mood swings
- restlessness
- use of alcohol or other drugs on a frequent basis
- headaches, dizziness, loss of appetite
- biting your nails, grinding your teeth, a dry mouth, feeling hot
- loss of appetite
- tightness in your neck, shoulders or back
- nausea, stomach cramps, diarrhea, constipation
- trouble sleeping

Consider these same symptoms as they relate to students. Do students get headaches before exams? Do young children cry or have temper tantrums during the first few weeks of school? Stress may be a contributor to these symptoms.

Coping with Stress

Examining your own reactions to stress can be insightful, as it is these reactions that children see—and copy. When you take a look at characteristics of your personality as they affect your levels of stress, you can see what children are learning from you. Often, your daily habits indicate how well you handle stress. For example, if you don't manage time well or eat a balanced diet, you may be prone to periods of time when even simple tasks become stressful. Exercise, on the other hand, is a daily habit that has several benefits—it keeps you healthy, gives you more energy and relieves stress.

Self-Assessment: Your Daily Habits and Stress

As you walk through this self-assessment, think about your daily routine. Consider whether any of your daily habits make it more difficult for you to handle stress. Then read through the questions again and see how many of your habits have a positive impact on your ability to handle stress.

As an educator, do you:

- Feel calm most of the time?
- Consider yourself a happy person?
- Think that others see you as a happy person?
- Have a good sense of humor?
- Associate with people who are happy and fulfilled?
- Feel excited about life?
- Keep a personal journal so that you have a way to process your feelings?

■ Delegate responsibility?

■ See a health professional if you are having trouble coping?

■ Get enough sleep?

■ Eat a balanced diet?

■ Exercise regularly?

Watch Out For...

■ Getting easily upset about minor problems such as spilling coffee or losing a pen.

■ Interrupting others because you can't wait for them to finish.

■ Rushing your speech.

■ Feeling impatient, which may lead you to eat too fast, resent waiting in line, get angry in heavy traffic.

■ Feeling so competitive that you hate to lose.

■ Taking work home with you.

■ Feeling short-tempered during the day and wondering why.

■ Feeling depressed.

■ Feeling stress about family events or holiday gatherings.

■ Consuming large amounts of caffeine.

Self-Assessment: Coping with Stress in the Classroom

Educators who deal well with stress and recognize what to do in stressful situations can be powerful models for children. Think about all the situations during a student's day that might be stressful. Then think about how you react to those situations. What can you do to teach students how to deal with their daily dilemmas? What do you model in the handling of your own everyday events?

As an educator, do you:

- Ever tell your students, "Bear with me today; I don't feel well," so they understand why you may be acting differently?

- Call on parents to help you in the classroom?

- Use stress-relieving techniques in the classroom such as deep breathing or closing your eyes and counting to 60?

- Laugh with your students?

- Talk with parents about the impact of stress on students?

Watch Out For...

- Being critical or sarcastic with students.

- Getting angry at students because they do not meet your expectations.

- Hurrying students because you want to move on to the next topic.

- Thinking about other things while students talk.

- Students who tend to be unusually competitive with one another.

- Coming down with numerous colds and flu viruses during the school year.

Stress Relievers

Adults have a responsibility not only to deal well with their own stress, but to help children deal with their stress, too. Stress for children often is not caused by the day-to-day activities of school and home but by being in situations where the options have been taken away or reduced.

Family Connection: Considerations for Parents

For most children, home is a "safe" environment. Home is the place where they receive nurturing, loving and support. After a hard day at school, home can help relieve the stress.

Parents play an enormous role in helping children learn to cope with stress. The parent who is always harried and who routinely hurries children in the morning not only sends them to school in a stressful state but teaches them that this is the way adults are supposed to act in the morning. The parent who helps children plan and organize the morning in order to leave for school in an unhurried fashion sends a different message about how adults behave in the morning.

Even special events or holidays can create stress for many people. Family gatherings, an upcoming wedding, the first few weeks of school, a new school, starting school without speaking English, making the basketball team, fear of violence at school—all of these can cause enough stress to send a child into a tailspin!

Children learn how to deal with stress from the adults—the models—in their lives. What are these adults' operational models? What personal characteristics do they demonstrate that children may emulate? Children observe and imitate what adults do, looking to them for examples of how to deal with stressful situations.

Parents can gain great insight into what their children are learning from them by examining their stress points and daily habits. The parent who laughs a lot is likely to raise children who can do the same. The parent who cannot deal with driving in rush-hour traffic or fixing dinner at night models to children that daily stress is inevitable and that routine tasks should be treated as a continuing series of crises.

The actions parents take are linked to their feelings and habits. How parents deal with stress and how they feel about themselves affect how they react to their children. A calm, well-rested parent may be much better equipped to deal with a morning when the milk is spilled, a backpack is torn and a mitten is missing than the parent who had only a few hours sleep, has already drunk several cups of coffee and is extremely agitated when the day is just beginning.

This self-assessment helps parents consider what they would like children to learn about daily routine and stress and how their personal habits might affect children's stress levels and ability to cope with stress.

(continued)

Modeling Healthy Behavior

Self-Assessment: Stress at Home

As a parent, do you:

- Think you are a happy person?
- Smile often?
- Enjoy being with children?
- Laugh often with children?
- Think children view you as happy and fun to be with?
- Establish a smooth morning routine?
- Have a friend (or spouse) to whom you can talk?
- Spend time with people who feel happy and fulfilled?
- Accept compliments well?
- Give compliments often?
- Exercise regularly?
- Get enough sleep?
- Eat a balanced breakfast?
- Maintain a healthy, comfortable body weight?
- Look forward to each day?

Watch Out For...

- Feeling easily rattled in the morning if someone loses a homework assignment or a lunch box.
- Rushing to work and school every morning.
- Rushed evenings, with many events or meetings to attend.
- Always feeling short on time.
- Interrupting others while they talk.
- Forgetting what you were going to say.
- Drinking a lot of coffee and colas.
- Losing your temper with children often.
- Feeling impatient if children are too slow or are not performing as well as you would like.
- Becoming upset when your children lose in sports or other games.
- Making fun of or criticizing children.

Skills for managing stress can be learned by children as well as adults. Decision making, goal setting, communication, problem solving and discipline are all activities that can help children—and adults—deal with daily life. Resilient children often have models in their lives who have learned skills for handling stress, including humor, social skills and problem-solving abilities.

Self-Assessment: Helping Students Relieve Stress

What can we do to help children relieve stress? In this self-assessment, you'll examine what you already do to help students relieve stress.

As an educator, do you:

- Know when students are under stress?

- See a pattern of stress behavior in some students?

- Talk to parents about stresses at school (e.g., a substitute teacher, an upcoming exam, a first school dance) so parents can help at home (or just know why a child might be anxious)?

- Have a school counselor available for students undergoing a crisis?

- Talk to students about what causes stress and how to handle it?

- Talk about the ways the body responds to stress?

- Use a comprehensive health education curriculum that talks about stress, decision making, problem solving, goal setting, etc.?

- Know what solutions to offer students experiencing problems?

- Talk about the importance of good nutrition and exercise and how healthy habits help the body deal with stressful situations?

- Recognize good behavior to help students feel good about their performance?

- Use stress-relieving activities such as taking a morning out of the classroom for a pleasant event?

Family Connection: Considerations for Parents

Parents can do a lot to help children relieve stress at home. Children look to their parents not only to show them how to relieve stress but also to assist them when help is needed. This self-assessment can help parents look at how they relive stress for their children.

Self-Assessment: Relieving Stress at Home

As a parent, do you:
- Think your children are happy?
- Know when children are under stress?
- Know children's stress signs?
- Know what helps children handle stress?
- Talk with children about events that may be stressful (for example, starting school, visiting relatives alone, having a new babysitter or taking a test)?
- Roleplay events that may cause stress (for example, riding the bus on the first day of school or trying out for the basketball team)?
- Try to manage stress during holidays and family vacations?
- Enjoy family time such as a night out at the movies or a family bike ride?
- Encourage family exercise to help manage stress?
- Offer balanced meals so children's nutritional requirements are met each day?
- Know if children have friends they can talk to?
- Talk often with children about school, friends, etc.?
- Spend one-on-one time with your children each day?
- Watch for signs of problems and seek professional help if needed?

Watch Out For...
- Letting children eat a lot of fast foods.
- Letting children skip meals.
- Planning so many activities for children that they don't have time to relax.

Setting Goals

The good news: Goal setting is not a genetically determined skill; it is learned behavior that begins in the early years. For adolescents, the many personal, educational and career decisions they are faced with can be overwhelming. Learning how to set—and meet—goals helps children deal with the daily stresses of growing up.

For young children, goal setting can be as simple as putting away their toys or making a date to play with friends after school. Older children deal with more complex goals. They may need to learn about who they are, their wants and needs, so they can better project what they want in the future. Their goals may include getting good grades to get into college, making the soccer team, or getting all of their home-work done so they can go to a dance. Some of these goals are long term, others are short term.

Parents and educators can help children learn how to set realistic goals, but not all adults are realistic in their goal setting. A parent who says, "I'm going back to college," "I'm going to write a book" or "I'm going to start a new business," but never does any of these things communicates that goals can be unrealistic and do not need to be met. An educator who tells the class, "We're going to have a pizza party when we finish this unit," but does not deliver the coveted reward not only disappoints the class, but tells them that reaching a goal may not bring the promised reward.

Some goals are unrealistic. A student who has no athletic ability may never make the starting squad of the basketball team. To let this student set such a goal only fosters the belief that goals are not to be met and diminishes self-esteem in the process. Other goals are not within the student's control. Young children living in households where a divorce is under way cannot set a goal of reuniting their parents by behaving better. This outcome is not within their power. No matter how good they are, the divorce may still occur.

Some people have difficulty setting any goals. If they have low self-esteem, the possibility of failing—not making the goal—may be paralyzing for even the simplest of daily goals. Striving to achieve a number of goals at the same time may be unrealistic as well. Someone who decides to lose 15 pounds, take up parachuting, finish a master's degree and coach the hockey team all at the same time may have difficulty with these goals and feel discouraged when they are not met.

Children need to learn that asking for help when working on goals is appropriate. If making the ski team means asking an adult to drive to the ski resort every day, then the child must do so to make the goal.

Short-term goals, and even long-term ones, can be adjusted without having to feel that the goal hasn't been met. If a goal of learning to tap dance by Christmas is missed because the teacher became ill and missed a month of lessons, then outside circumstances have altered the time frame for meeting the goal. But the goal of learning the skill is still attainable.

Self-Assessment: Modeling Goal Setting at School

Children take their cues from models in their lives when it comes to setting goals. What kind of goal-setting behavior do you think students learn from you? Do they see you as someone who sets a realistic goal and meets it? Or do they see you as someone who constantly sets goals that have no possibility of being reached? Based on your goal-setting modeling, what kinds of habits do you think your students possess now—and will possess when they are adults?

In the next self-assessment, you can check your own goal setting—and goal reaching. By reflecting on your own habits, you can better perceive what you are modeling for students.

As an educator, do you:

■ Think you set realistic goals?

■ Reach your own goals?

■ Encourage others to reach their goals?

■ Value who you are and the goals you have met in your life?

■ Realize the importance of goal setting both for you and for students?

Watch Out For...

■ Setting too many goals at one time.

■ Procrastinating because you cannot create a goal or reach the goal.

■ Making New Years' resolutions that you know you won't keep.

■ Wondering why you don't reach goals you set.

■ Feeling that you are a failure because you can't reach goals.

■ Criticizing others for setting goals.

■ Criticizing others for reaching or not reaching goals.

Self-Assessment: Goal Setting in the Classroom

Goal setting is a major component of any classroom. The first-grade students who read books to earn a pizza party learn that setting a goal—and reaching it—feels good. The high school student who wants to get an A in English sets a goal of completing all assignments and achieving a score of at least 90 percent on all of them.

Educators can have a significant amount of influence over how students learn to set goals. A teacher who says, "Please finish all of your math before going to lunch," gives students a goal to reach. A teacher who says, "Please finish all of your math, reading and science before lunch," when this may be impossible for most students, forces students to aim for a goal that is unattainable.

Explore how you work with students when it comes to goal setting. These patterns of setting and reaching goals are crucial habits for students, and you are pivotal in what students learn about goal setting.

Family Connection: Considerations for Parents

Parents are the first models of goal setting for children. Toddlers who learn they must eat their snack before getting down from the table learn to set a simple goal. Children not only see parents setting and reaching their own goals but are aided in the goal-setting process by the models in their lives. The following self-assessment helps parents explore how they aid their children in learning goal-setting skills.

Self-Assessment: Modeling Goal Setting at Home

As a parent, do you:
- Understand the difference between short-term and long-term goals?
- Help children learn to set both short-term and long-term goals?
- Help children set goals they can reach?
- Offer rewards when goals are met and come through with promised rewards?
- Compliment children as they make steps toward reaching a goal?
- Talk to children about goals they might not reach?
- Help children work through the consequences of not meeting a goal?
- Think your children feel good when they reach goals?
- Think your children will grow up with good goal-setting skills?

Watch Out For...
- Making it hard for children to set goals.
- Making it harder for children to reach goals because you don't have time to help them.
- Criticizing children for not meeting a goal.

As an educator, do you:

■ Clearly define your expectations for students?

■ Set clear and specific goals for yourself and students?

■ Help students work toward their goals?

■ Notice when students are not meeting goals and discuss this with them?

- Discuss goal setting with students and talk about short-term and long-term goals?

- Roleplay with students about goal setting?

- Help students work toward group goals as well as individual ones?

- Reward students when they make their goals?

- Make sure that you deliver what you promise?

- Enjoy helping students meet goals?

Watch Out For...

- Being sarcastic or critical if students don't reach a goal.

- Discouraging students from reaching goals because introducing needed skills takes too much of your time.

Problem Solving and Decision Making

Learning to make decisions is an important part of growing up. Some decisions, such as deciding to eat breakfast every day or to go to bed in time to get a good night's sleep, create habits. Home and classroom settings encourage group decision making and problem solving. When children learn at a young age that problems can be solved, they are better equipped to handle bigger problems—drugs, bullies, difficult teachers—when they approach adolescence.

A number of factors influence decision making, including personal skills, experience, beliefs and values, as well as other internal or external pressures. Very young children who do not understand the consequences of running into the street make that decision without the benefit of experience. Teenagers who want to attend a party when parents have forbidden it face social pressure from friends for not attending, but also understand the consequences of deciding to disobey. Those consequences may not matter as much as friends' approval, and they may go to the party anyway.

Peer pressure often directly conflicts with parents' desires. Even with consistent demands from adults, children may still be greatly affected by social pressures.

Children with low self-esteem are more likely to have difficulty with problem solving and decision making. Young children who have few friends may choose to hit or kick other children to get attention. The decision to use these tactics to solve the problem is fueled by poor self-esteem. Such children badly want friends and have no idea how to act like a friend, so they will try anything to reach their goal.

Adults both model decision making and problem solving and can work with children to help them develop and improve these skills. Children like to feel that they can make their own decisions. As they make more and more choices, they learn about the consequences—both good and bad—of their decisions and begin to feel that they are more in control of their lives.

Self-Assessment: Your Decision-Making Foundation

Checking your own decision-making abilities gives you clues to what students are learning from you. If making decisions is very difficult for you, or if it's hard for you to accept the consequences of your choices, students will assume that this is acceptable decision-making behavior. This self-assessment helps you take stock of your own decision-making foundation.

As an educator, do you:

- Take the time to solve problems in a logical manner?
- Easily make decisions?
- Think that others view you as a decisive person?

- Follow through on decisions?
- Understand the consequences of your decisions and readily accept them?

Watch Out For...

- Worrying about the outcome of your decisions.
- Brooding over bad decisions.
- Feeling that every day is an endless stream of decisions and problems.
- Avoiding making decisions.
- Worrying that others will think you're stupid if you make a mistake.
- Giving up if you can't finish something and labeling yourself a failure.
- Criticizing others for their decisions.

Self-Assessment: Decision Making in the Classroom

Students practice making decisions in the classroom every day. Young students may choose which learning center to visit. Older students choose to get to class on time, eat lunch with certain friends or take their band instruments home for practice sessions.

The decisions educators make in the classroom are observed. These observations can assist students with solving their own problems and making their own decisions. Think about students' perception of you as a decision maker, as well as how you implement decision-making activities in the classroom.

As an educator, do you:

- Let students see some of the daily decisions you make?
- Let students see you solve problems?
- Include students in solving problems?
- Engage small or large groups in solving problems?
- Help students understand the consequences of making decisions?
- Roleplay with students on problem solving and decision making?
- Compliment students on their decisions?
- Talk with parents about decision making and problem solving?
- Use a health education curriculum that includes decision-making and problem-solving units?
- Offer support to students when they are having difficulty with problem solving?
- Know when students in your class are making poor decisions?
- Let students experience the consequences of their decisions? (For example, if students must complete an assignment before recess, do you support your statement by keeping in students who have decided not to complete the work?)
- Get involved in group decision making with other school staff?
- Help students learn from their mistakes?
- Let students make decisions about their day, such as choosing to read, work on a math project or help another student?

Watch Out For...

- Rushing students into making decisions.
- Saying things such as "That was a bad decision. Look what you've done."

Family Connection: Considerations for Parents

Parents can evaluate how they model decision making at home. Do they encourage children to take risks when making decisions? Will children be chastised if they make a wrong choice? Are children able to work through problems on their own? The following self-assessment can assist parents in evaluating the decision-making skills they model for their children.

Self-Assessment: Decision Making at Home

As a parent, do you:
- Think your children will make good choices as they grow up?
- Let children know that adults make mistakes?
- Ask children for help in making decisions?
- Make some decisions together as a family (for example, where to vacation or how to celebrate a birthday)?
- Think children see you as a strong decision maker?
- Offer children choices so they can make decisions?
- Help children understand the consequences of their decisions?
- Think your children make good decisions?
- Help children if they are unhappy with their decisions?
- Understand how peer pressure may affect children's decisions?

Watch Out For...
- Criticizing children for making bad decisions.
- Telling children they can't make a decision because they don't know how.
- Worrying about how children will react to your decisions.

Communication

Communication with students, parents, colleagues, friends and family is part of everyday life. Even infants communicate with their parents by crying and smiling—clear signs of their feelings. Preschoolers ask for a glass of juice, comment on the day at the playground or talk to a friend. Older students communicate with their teachers about their studies and with their peers about their daily lives.

Knowing how to communicate affects our level of self-esteem and determines the quality of our relationships. Good communication skills are a necessity—they open the door to learning about others and to expressing our own feelings. Many people can relate a classic failure-to-communicate story, in which one party assumed one thing while the other party saw the same issue in an entirely different way. The two people didn't communicate, and each became angry or frustrated.

For educators, knowing how to communicate is vital. How can students learn if an educator cannot express the ideas? While educators are communicating to students, students are learning more than just the ideas at hand. They are learning how to communicate. Educators show students how to talk about ideas, listen, ask questions, participate, include others in discussion and have their thoughts acknowledged.

Children who do not know how to communicate often cannot find constructive ways to release the anger, frustration or even good feelings that are inside. This inability to express emotions can lower self-esteem and result in social isolation. Children who do not have the social skills that let them become part of a group of friends often lack communication skills.

The stresses of everyday life can build up in children who cannot communicate their feelings. If children can't talk about the wet socks inside their boots, tell the coach that they forgot the permission slip for the upcoming meet, or discuss their fears about making an oral book report, they will feel additional stress.

Communication skills begin at the earliest development stages and continue to be refined through adulthood. Adults are important models of communication skills. Talking—and listening—to children helps them become involved and learn how to communicate.

Self-Assessment: Your Communication Skills

In this self-assessment, you can reflect on your communication skills. Are you able to talk easily about your feelings, or do you bottle them up inside? Can you go into a social setting and easily converse with people you do not know? Do you have friends and family with whom you can talk about everyday occurrences? Think about how you routinely communicate and what children learn as you talk about the weather, the day at school or problems with friends.

As an educator, do you:

- Feel comfortable talking about your feelings?

- Consider yourself a good listener?

- Make eye contact when you speak?

- Know how to say no and mean it?

- Give clear and specific directions?

- Consider yourself a good communicator?

- Feel comfortable talking on the phone?

- Occasionally write letters to friends?

- Feel comfortable showing anger?

- Have a good sense of humor?

Self-Assessment: Communication in the Classroom

Communication is an important part of the school day. Students learn many communication skills from educators as they discover how to talk to teachers or friends. Do students see you as someone they can talk to? Do you listen to students and truly understand what they have to say? Do you help students learn how to communicate? Do students leave your classroom with improved communication skills?

Family Connection: Considerations for Parents

Many communication skills are learned at home. Parents can consider the communication skills they would like their children to possess. Are these skills modeled and practiced in the home? This self-assessment helps parents evaluate the communication skills and practices they model for their children.

Self-Assessment: Communication at Home

As a parent, do you:
- Let children hear you talking to other adults?
- Think what children say is important?
- Talk often with your children's teachers about school activities and how your children are doing?
- Teach children to express their anger in ways that don't hurt themselves or others?
- Ask questions about your children's day every day?
- Understand what children are talking about?
- Have family discussions, perhaps around the dinner table?
- Spend one-on-one time daily with your children (for example, reading to them)?
- Think your children can talk to you about their problems?
- Understand children's feelings?
- Give clear directions when you ask children to clean up the kitchen or put away their toys?
- Enjoy listening to children talk to their friends?
- Ask questions that require more than yes or no answers?
- Teach children how to write thank-you notes or talk on the telephone?
- Laugh with children instead of at them?
- Let children cry when they need to?

Watch Out For...
- Making fun of children.
- Scolding children for crying.
- Discounting children's feelings.

As an educator, do you:

- Let students see you talking not only to them, but to other adults?

- Bring other adults such as administrators, parents or other teachers into your classroom to talk with students?

- Communicate often with parents?

- Try to avoid lecturing and include students in discussions?

- Know how much time you spend lecturing and how much time you allow for discussion?

- Use hands-on activities to help students express ideas?

- Observe what students are feeling?

- Seek students out when you sense they are stressed and try to help them communicate?

- Consider yourself someone students can talk to?

- Encourage all students to participate in the classroom?

- Find ways to encourage quiet students to communicate?

- Let students share ideas with each other?

- Listen to what students have to say?

- Ask questions that help students open up?

- Feel students understand what you say?

Discipline and Consequences

In learning how to deal with stress, make decisions, solve problems and communicate, children will make mistakes. A student who is upset because he got a low grade on a test but who talks to the teacher about the assignment and how to do better next time uses and reinforces good communication skills. The student who tears up the paper and storms out of the room has not yet learned the appropriate skills to deal with such issues.

We want children to learn from their decisions and so boost their self-esteem. The educator who acknowledges good behavior with positive comments helps children feel that they can make decisions they will feel good about. Berating children for leaving homework at home will tell them that when they make a mistake, they should feel bad. They will learn to bring in the homework not because they want to do well, but because they don't want to be yelled at.

There are two ways of dealing with children when they make mistakes or behave badly: punishing them or allowing them to experience the consequences of their actions. Students who forget their homework can learn either by being punished—yelled at—or by experiencing the consequences—having their grades lowered.

When students who make a mistake in a math problem while writing it on the board are laughed at or berated, they may be unwilling to take such risks in the future. On the other hand, if teachers point out such errors and offer suggestions to students to correct the mistakes, praising students for thinking through the equation, they teach that making a mistake can be a positive experience.

Discipline and guidelines help children know where the boundaries are. Learning that they cannot go on a field trip because they forgot the permission slip helps students learn to be responsible for their actions. A well-disciplined class is one that clearly knows what the teacher expects and works to meet those expectations because of the rewards that come with those accomplishments.

Self-Assessment: Modeling Discipline and Consequences

Students learn a great deal about discipline from educators. As you work through the next self-assessment, think about the boundaries you establish in your classroom and the kinds of lessons these boundaries are providing students. What are you modeling to students when you expect and reward responsible behavior? What kinds of behavior habits are students learning from you?

As an educator, do you:

■ Have clearly defined classroom rules?

■ Repeat those rules regularly?

■ Explain why the rules are important?

■ Inform parents of classroom rules?

■ Communicate with parents about consequences when rules are broken?

■ Have high expectations for students?

■ Give students responsibilities?

■ Assign tasks to students on a rotating basis so everyone gets a chance to take part?

■ Provide support, if needed, when tasks are being completed?

■ Compliment students who successfully complete assignments?

■ Act consistently when more than one student makes the same mistake?

■ Consider your class to be well disciplined?

■ Expect responsible and respectful behavior from students?

■ Clearly express your displeasure with inappropriate behavior?

■ Try to let consequences rather than punishment encourage good behavior?

■ Include students in establishing consequences?

■ Follow through with consequences?

■ Predict when some students will make mistakes or misbehave and present solutions as soon as possible?

Watch Out For...

- ■ Criticizing students while they complete assignments.

- ■ Feeling you always have to be right to save face with your students.

Family Connection: Considerations for Parents

Parents may want to review how they discipline their children at home. Does the family foster a sense of responsibility among all family members? If parents look into the future to see their children as parents, will their grandchildren grow up to be responsible, learning from their parents what their grandparents are modeling today?

The following self-assessment assists parents in forming family guidelines about discipline.

Self-Assessment: Discipline at Home

As a parent, do you:

- • Expect children to be courteous, respectful and responsible?
- • Speak clearly when you give children directions?
- • Have clear and consistent rules so children know what is expected?
- • Give children regular family jobs to do?
- • Notice both good and bad behavior?
- • Think your children are well behaved?

Watch Out For...

- • Making threats you don't mean.
- • Yelling before you think about what you're saying.
- • Punishing instead of letting children experience the consequences of their actions.
- • Using punishment that doesn't relate to the behavior (for example, not letting a child play with friends because she left her backpack at school).
- • Making fun of children when they make mistakes.

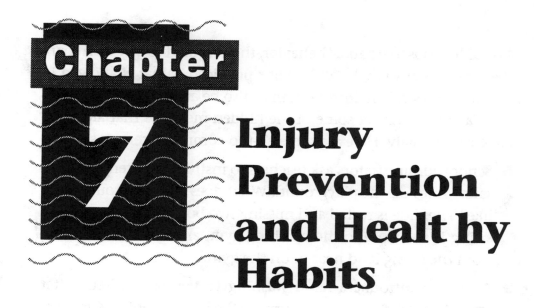

Chapter 7

Injury Prevention and Healthy Habits

KEEPING CHILDREN HEALTHY and safe means helping them to acquire the awareness, knowledge and skills they need to take good care of themselves—and providing them with opportunities to practice what they've learned in the classroom.

Good health and safety habits are preventive strategies, and their benefits may not be obvious right away. Unfortunately, when these habits are not practiced, their usefulness can be fully appreciated. Because prevention is a hard concept for children and adolescents to absorb, these behaviors must be learned at an early age so that they become habits—behaviors that are automatic.

The school setting is only one environment where children can practice the healthy behaviors they have learned. Most opportunities to practice these behaviors are in the community, among family and friends. What children see—what is modeled to them—in these environments has a significant influence on their perception of what is important and what constitutes "adult" behavior, and on their likelihood of putting this behavior into routine practice.

As children observe adults' behavior, they are alert to any discrepancies between what's taught and what's practiced. What is allowed in the social or physical environment may also be at odds with messages that are taught. Consider some of the hidden messages that are modeled to children daily. Here are some all-too-common scenarios:

- School administrators ask teachers to instruct children to follow safety rules on the playground. What does the playground look like? The slide is rusted and missing two bolts on a support. The swing is too close to the climbing gym, and children jumping from the swing land near or on the gym.

- A teacher introduces hand washing to young children. After several weeks, the teacher returns to the habit of not washing his hands in front of the children.

- A parent constantly reminds children to fasten their safety belts, but she neglects to fasten her own.

In each of these examples, the behaviors that adults attempt to teach are contradicted by what they model. Children receive mixed messages, and often it is the modeled message that is remembered, rather than the principle that was taught.

Threats to Children's Health and Safety

The leading cause of death among children and youth is unintentional injury. Historically, this cause has been mislabeled as "accidents," implying that events were random or uncontrollable. Now public health leaders discourage the use of this term, since it can lead people to assume that injuries are not preventable. Many of them are.

For instance, most automobile crashes resulting in death involve drivers who have been drinking. Driving at high speeds and failing to use safety belts are also causes of injury and death. For children, major causes of death include drowning and household fires. Other injuries are the result of falls, poisonings and unsafe play equipment or activities. As Table 1 shows, younger children and youth have different experiences, as do girls and boys.

Table 1

Leading Causes of Death (U.S.),Children and Youth Ages 5–24

	Rate/100,000 Population					
	Age 5–14			Age 15–24		
Cause	All	Males	Females	All	Males	Females
All causes	25.8	30.9	20.4	102.1	151.0	52.1
All injury (% motor vehicle)	12.2 (57.4)	15.7 (55.4)	8.4 (61.9)	49.5 (77.8)	75.1 (75.4)	23.3 (86.3)
Homicide	1.3	1.5	1.1	15.4	24.7	6.0
Suicide	0.7	1.0	0.7	13.2	21.9	4.2
Malignant neoplasms (cancers)	3.2	3.6	2.7	5.1	5.9	4.2
Heart disease	0.9	1.1	0.8	2.9	3.8	2.1
Congenital anomalies	1.4	1.6	1.3	1.3	1.4	1.1
HIV/AIDS	—	—		1.4	2.4	0.5

Source: U.S. Department of Health and Human Services. 1988. *National Center for Health Statistics: Annual Report.* Washington, DC.

While children now experience fewer deaths from infectious diseases, these are still important threats to children's health and are responsible for many absences from school. Immunizations have made a big impact on many childhood diseases, such as polio, diphtheria and whooping cough, but some disturbing trends have begun to change this picture. Many children are not being immunized at a young enough age. Areas that have higher numbers of immigrants also have increasing rates of TB and other diseases such as smallpox.

The physical and social environments of children are also significant. An alarming number of children under 18 years of age—1.2 million in 1989—are living in poverty. African-American or Latino children are three times more likely to live in poverty than White children. Poverty puts children's health and safety in jeopardy, both long term and in the course of daily living.

Most health problems experienced by youth don't result in immediate death and may take many years to have a serious impact. Many experts agree that a better measure of the health status of youth is the presence or absence of health-compromising behaviors.

Unhealthy or unsafe behaviors, such as smoking, early and unprotected sexual intercourse, or alcohol and other drug use, when started at a young age, can eventually cause illness, disability or death. These behaviors include those that result in unintentional and intentional injuries, for example, failure to use protective devices such as safety belts or bicycle helmets, fighting and violence, youth gang activities and suicide.

Injury Prevention and Safety

Although most educators include some injury prevention in their curriculum, modeling this concept is an important component of teaching. Checking our everyday habits can indicate how safety conscious we are and suggest areas for improvement.

Self-Assessment: Modeling Safe Actions at School

Children learn a great deal from what we do, and how we model safety habits in the classroom may be an area that educators do not think about enough. Children are always watching—and learning—from what we model. The safety consciousness and injury prevention habits you demonstrate in the classroom may well become the habits students adopt as their own. How do you rate yourself on these safety habits? Where could you improve?

As an educator, do you:

- Generally know safety rules?

- Know emergency numbers for fire, ambulance, police?

- Follow traffic rules when walking with students (cross in the crosswalk, cross with the light, walk on the sidewalk, look both ways before crossing, etc.)?

- Spend time at the beginning of each school year talking about safety in your classroom, playground, etc.?

- Walk through the playground from time to time to check for safety?

- Talk about traffic safety, fire safety and bike safety with your students?

- Know what safety rules your school considers important?

- Check that areas of the school receiving heavy traffic are safe and free of water or obstacles (e.g., areas around lockers, hallways, cafeteria or gymnasium)?

- Talk about safety issues in staff meetings?

- Consider your school a safe place?

- Know if the crosswalks in front of your school are monitored?

- Know if areas where buses arrive are safe?

- Know what kinds of chemicals might be used in science, art or shop classes and if students are instructed in how to use these chemicals?

■ Notice if children wear reflective material if they arrive at school before daylight?

Watch Out For...

■ Trying to reach something in the classroom by standing on a desk or chair.

■ Overloading the electrical outlets in the classroom.

Family Connection: Considerations for Parents

Parents can reflect on their safety habits to see what children are learning from them. Consider what children learn when parents install a smoke detector in the house or insist on using crosswalks and waiting for the light to change. The attitudes and habits parents have about safety are observed by children every day.

Self-Assessment: Safety Habits at Home

As a parent, do you:

- Think about safety each day?
- Teach your children the emergency numbers to call and post them for all family members to see?
- Teach children to be safe in the kitchen by taking safe actions yourself (for example, using knives correctly, keeping pan handles turned away from the edge of the stove, being careful with hot oils, watching children as they cook for themselves, carrying hot dishes correctly)?
- Give baby sitters information about safety?
- Keep stairways free of clutter?
- Store dangerous chemicals safely?
- Use reflective material on backpacks and clothing used in the dark?
- Know if your children follow rules for pedestrian safety (cross at crosswalks, walk on sidewalks, use crossing guards, etc.)?
- Know if the playground at your children's school is safe?
- Know if your children's school has a safety committee?
- Know what kinds of injury prevention skills are taught at your children's school?

(continued)

Watch Out For...

- Ignoring safety rules "just this once."
- Thinking that "it won't happen to me."
- Criticizing other parents for being safety conscious.
- Taking unsafe actions (such as standing on the kitchen counter to reach something).
- Overloading electrical outlets.
- Being "too busy" to fix unsafe things around your home.
- Asking children to wear protective items such as safety belts or bicycle helmets but not wearing them yourself.
- Teasing children about the way they look in safety equipment.
- Criticizing the school for requiring safety equipment.

Self-Assessment: Modeling Safe Driving Behaviors

Automobile crashes are a primary cause of childhood injury and death. Safe behaviors in the car are of paramount importance. Adults must show children that they respect and observe the rules for safe driving and safe behaviors in the car.

As an educator, do you:

■ Always wear your safety belt?

■ Know if students see you driving to school?

■ Regularly maintain or check the safety of your car?

■ Obey the speed limit and follow basic rules of the road?

■ Talk about safe driving with students?

■ Demonstrate respect for the work that police and highway patrol officers do to keep roadways safe?

■ Never drive after drinking and refuse to ride with anyone who does?

Family Connection: Considerations for Parents

Parents are the adults children have the most opportunities to watch. Their driving habits are visible every time a child gets in the car. Do parents consider themselves safe drivers? Do they have room for improvement in what they model to their children? The following self-assessment helps parents evaluate their modeling of safe behaviors in the car.

Self-Assessment: Driving Safely

As a parent, do you:

- Always wear your safety belt and insist that children wear theirs?
- Check the safety of your car?
- Obey the speed limit and follow basic rules of the road?
- Show respect for the work that police and highway patrol officers do to keep roadways safe?
- Allow joggers or bicyclists plenty of room on the road?
- Never drive after drinking and refuse to ride with anyone who does?

Watch Out For...

- Making negative comments about how others drive.
- Criticizing others for driving at the speed limit.
- Taking risks while you drive (for example, driving too fast, passing on the shoulder).
- Saying things such as "Uh oh, there's a cop. I'd better slow down."

Self-Assessment: Modeling Safety in Sports

Physical education teachers and coaches are in a unique position to model injury prevention habits. How these teachers address safety has an impact on other teachers, parents and students. However, all educators can benefit from an assessment of their safety behaviors in the area of sports and recreation.

Sports Nutrition

Dear Family:

If your children are involved in sports, you need to understand what kinds of foods children need both at mealtimes and as snacks before training and at games and meets. Good choices include:

- foods high in complex carbohydrates, such as fruits, vegetables and whole grains
- bananas and oranges
- performance drinks or water

These foods help supply the nutrients that are used during a workout.

Parents and coaching staff can work together to help children learn that good nutrition is important to being good athletes. When you encourage the athletes in your family to eat healthy meals, you help establish lifelong patterns of healthy eating.

The following self-assessment looks at what you know about sports nutrition and how you model or encourage healthy eating habits. You don't need to write out answers to these questions. Just be honest with yourself. Remember, there is no one "right" way to behave, but what you learn from this self-assessment may help you do some things differently.

Self-Assessment: Sports Nutrition at Home

As a parent, do you:

- Understand what sports nutrition is?
- Know if your children's coach talks about sports nutrition with students?
- Ask the coach to provide information on sports nutrition?
- Know what kinds of food children need at meals and snacks?
- Plan to meet the nutritional needs of children?
- Provide snacks that offer complex carbohydrates and protein before and after training?
- Ask children to help shop and prepare food?

Watch Out For...

- Letting a child's coach suggest that the child lose weight.
- Encouraging children to lose weight quickly before a sporting event.

Fitness

Dear Family:

Parents are important models of fitness. What you do at home can inspire children to include fitness in their daily lives. Children look at your fitness habits and attitudes every day. Does your family do things together such as skiing, biking or walking? Do children see that fitness is a family activity that everyone enjoys?

Many parents may not know much about the school program of physical education (PE). But you are a very important part of these programs. Your personal commitment to overall fitness and your support of the school PE program tell children that fitness is important.

The following self-assessment can help you examine family attitudes toward fitness. It may also encourage you to find out more about the school's PE program. You don't need to write out answers to these questions. Just be honest with yourself. Remember, there is no one "right" way to behave, but what you learn from this self-assessment may help you do some things differently.

Self-Assessment: Fitness at Home

Family Fitness

As a parent, do you:

- Promote fitness and exercise at home?
- Exercise regularly?
- Take part in lifetime fitness activities such as walking, swimming, biking or tennis?
- Make time for family activities such as walking, biking, swimming or skiing?
- Let children see you as an active person?
- Think your children will grow up to be active and fit if they follow in your footsteps?
- Wear the right clothing for your fitness activities?

Watch Out For...

- Having fitness equipment you don't use.
- Saying, "I'll start exercising tomorrow."

School Fitness

As a parent, do you:

- Understand the PE program in your children's school?

(continued)

- Know how often students have PE?
- Know if all grade levels have PE?
- Know how children are graded in PE?
- Talk to the PE teacher during parent/teacher conferences?
- Get information on fitness from the school?
- Know if children's teachers take part in PE classes or watch from the sidelines?
- Talk with children about PE classes?
- Make sure children have the exercise clothing or shoes they need?
- Know if fitness testing is used in the school?
- Understand that PE is important to children's health?
- See educators actively involved in fitness activities such as running or walking?
- Help children take part in after-school sports?
- Help children stay fit?
- Get involved with children's sports (for example, attend events or parent meetings, offer to help the coach)?

Messages About Smoking

Dear Family:

Many nonsmokers in the United States are worried about health problems related to tobacco smoke. Nonsmokers breathe two kinds of smoke when they are around smokers—sidestream smoke and secondhand smoke. Sidestream smoke is the smoke from the tip of a burning cigarette or cigar; secondhand smoke is the smoke the smoker exhales. Both of these kinds of smoke affect nonsmokers.

Experts estimate that almost half the children in the United States live in families where someone smokes. Children with asthma or other breathing problems are even more at risk when they live in households with smokers.

Trying to keep your home smoke free shows children that you want to keep them healthy. If you smoke, you may decide to smoke outside or to smoke only in rooms that are well-ventilated. You may also want to ask visitors to your home who smoke to smoke only in certain places.

When your family visits other homes where smokers live, can you ask the smokers not to smoke while your children are there? Special events for children, such as birthday parties or scout meetings, should also have no-smoking rules.

Think about the messages you send children about tobacco use. Do children see that you try to keep cigarette smoke away from them? If your children grow up with your habits and attitudes about smoking, will they be smokers or nonsmokers?

You don't need to write out answers to these questions. Just be honest with yourself. Remember, there is no one "right" way to behave, but what you learn from this self-assessment may help you do some things differently.

Self-Assessment: Messages About Smoking at Home

As a parent, do you:

- Keep your home smoke free?
- Keep parts of your home (such as children's bedrooms) smoke free?
- Ask guests to smoke outside?
- Ask others not to smoke around your family?
- Ask to be seated in nonsmoking sections in restaurants?
- Talk about tobacco advertising with your children?
- Know if your children's school has a smoke-free policy?
- Work for a smoke-free school?
- Know if your school teaches children about the dangers of tobacco use?

(continued)

- Offer to help at school when children are learning about preventing the use of tobacco?
- Encourage friends or family to quit smoking?
- Know if parents of your children's friends smoke when your child visits?
- Tell children about health problems related to smoking?

Watch Out For...

- Keeping cigarettes where children can see them.
- Buying cigarettes in front of children.
- Offering cigarettes to others.
- Smoking in front of children.
- Sending children to buy cigarettes.

Messages About Alcohol

Dear Family:

Children need to know that alcohol and other drugs are dangerous to their health. Thus, adults must not only speak clearly on this subject, but must act clearly as well. We give children confusing messages when we tell them to avoid these drugs but use them ourselves.

You influence your children's beliefs about drinking and drug use. Children who grow up with little exposure to alcohol are less likely to have problems with all kinds of drug use. Family situations that may be more likely to lead to problem drinking include:

- Unclear and inconsistent drinking practices.
- One parent favors drinking and the other opposes it.
- Standards for drinking are different for men and women.

As you look at the models you offer related to alcohol, think about your own habits and attitudes. Do children often see alcohol in the home? Do they observe adults who are intoxicated? What do children think when you offer guests a drink? Do the attitudes you model support what you want for your children?

You don't need to write out answers to these questions. Just be honest with yourself. Remember, there is no one "right" way to behave, but what you learn from this self-assessment may help you do some things differently.

Self-Assessment: Messages About Alcohol at Home

As a parent, do you:

- Make it clear that use of too much alcohol is not acceptable?
- Avoid pressuring people to drink alcohol?
- Make it clear that drinking too much is not funny?
- Offer guests non-alcoholic drinks as well as alcoholic drinks?
- Never let guests drive home after drinking?

Watch Out For...

- Drinking alcohol as a way to escape problems.
- Drinking alcohol or using other drugs after work because you had a bad day.
- Drinking to intoxication.
- Allowing children to observe intoxicated adults.
- Leaving liquor bottles out for children to see or obtain.
- Always including alcohol in family events, parties or celebrations.
- Rewarding children with an alcoholic drink for a special occasion.
- Buying alcohol when children are present.

Stress

Dear Family:

Stress is the feeling of being under pressure. This pressure affects children and adults in many different ways. Stress may be caused by a job change, a new baby or a divorce.

But it is not just major life events that trigger stress. Research now shows that even daily stresses can be hard for some people to handle. Daily hassles such as oversleeping, bouncing a check or forgetting to put out the garbage can add up.

Even special events or holidays can create stress for many people. Family gatherings, an upcoming wedding, starting school, making the basketball team, fear of violence at school—all of these can cause enough stress to send a child into a tailspin!

For most children, home is a "safe" place. Home is where they receive love and support. Home can help relieve the stress of a hard day at school. Children learn how to deal with stress from the adults—the models—in their lives. They look to us for examples of how to deal with stress. What do you model for children in this area?

Think about your daily habits and things that cause you stress. If you laugh a lot, your children are likely to do the same. If you cannot deal with driving in rush-hour traffic, you may be teaching children that daily stress can't be avoided. If you feel stress about fixing dinner at night, children may learn that routine tasks should be treated as problems.

How you deal with stress and how you feel about yourself affect how you act with your children. Consider what you would like children to learn about daily routine and stress. How do your personal habits affect children's stress levels and their ability to cope with stress?

You don't need to write out answers to these questions. Just be honest with yourself. Remember, there is no one "right" way to behave, but what you learn from this self-assessment may help you do some things differently.

Self-Assessment: Stress at Home

As a parent, do you:
- Think you are a happy person?
- Smile often?
- Enjoy being with children?
- Laugh often with children?
- Think children view you as happy and fun to be with?
- Establish a smooth morning routine?
- Have a friend (or spouse) to whom you can talk?

(continued)

- Spend time with people who feel happy and fulfilled?
- Accept compliments well?
- Give compliments often?
- Exercise regularly?
- Get enough sleep?
- Eat a balanced breakfast?
- Maintain a healthy, comfortable body weight?
- Look forward to each day?

Watch Out For...

- Feeling easily rattled in the morning if someone loses a homework assignment or a lunch box.
- Rushing to work and school every morning.
- Rushed evenings, with many events or meetings to attend.
- Always feeling short on time.
- Interrupting others while they talk.
- Forgetting what you were going to say.
- Drinking a lot of coffee and colas.
- Losing your temper with children often.
- Feeling impatient if children are too slow or are not performing as well as you would like.
- Becoming upset when your children lose in sports or other games.
- Making fun of or criticizing children.

Relieving Stress

Dear Family:

Parents can help children learn to handle stress. Show children how to relieve stress and offer your help when they need it. This self-assessment lets you look at how you help children relieve stress.

You don't need to write out answers to these questions. Just be honest with yourself. Remember, there is no one "right" way to behave, but what you learn from this self-assessment may help you do some things differently.

Self-Assessment: Relieving Stress at Home

As a parent, do you:

- Think your children are happy?
- Know when children are under stress?
- Know children's stress signs?
- Know what helps children handle stress?
- Talk with children about events that may be stressful (for example, starting a new school, visiting relatives by themselves, having a new babysitter or taking a test)?
- Roleplay events that may cause stress (for example, riding the bus on the first day of school or trying out for the basketball team)?
- Try to manage stress during holidays and family vacations?
- Enjoy family time such as a night out at the movies or a family bike ride?
- Encourage family exercise to help manage stress?
- Offer balanced meals so children get the healthy foods they need each day?
- Know if children have friends they can talk to?
- Talk often with children about school, friends, etc.?
- Spend one-on-one time with your children each day?
- Watch for signs of problems and seek professional help if needed?

Watch Out For...
- Letting children eat a lot of fast foods.
- Letting children skip meals.
- Planning so many activities for children that they don't have time to relax.

Goal Setting

Dear Family:

Learning how to set and meet goals helps children deal with the daily stresses of growing up. For young children, goal setting can be as simple as putting away their toys. As children get a little older, goal setting may involve activities such as making a date to play with friends after school.

Older children deal with more complex goals. Their goals may include making a sports team, getting all their homework done so they can do something else, or getting good grades. Some goals are short term—they can be met in a few days or a few weeks. Other goals are long term—they may take many days or even years to reach.

Parents are the first models of goal setting for children. Toddlers who learn they must eat their snack before they get down from the table learn to set a simple goal. When children see parents setting and reaching goals, they learn about the goal-setting process.

The following self-assessment helps you explore how you help children learn to set goals. You don't need to write out answers to these questions. Just be honest with yourself. Remember, there is no one "right" way to behave, but what you learn from this self-assessment may help you do some things differently.

Self-Assessment: Modeling Goal Setting at Home

As a parent, do you:

- Understand the difference between short-term and long-term goals?
- Help children learn to set both short-term and long-term goals?
- Help children set goals they can reach?
- Offer rewards when goals are met and come through with promised rewards?
- Compliment children as they make steps toward reaching a goal?
- Talk to children about goals they might not reach?
- Help children work through the consequences of not meeting a goal?
- Think your children feel good when they reach goals?
- Think your children will grow up with good goal-setting skills?

Watch Out For...

- Making it hard for children to set goals.
- Making it harder for children to reach goals because you don't have time to help them.
- Criticizing children for not meeting a goal.

Decision Making

Dear Family:

Learning to make decisions is an important part of growing up. Children like to feel that they can make their own decisions. As children make more and more choices, they learn about the consequences, both good and bad, of their decisions. They also begin to feel that they are more in control of their lives.

Think about how you model decision making at home. Do you encourage children to take some chances when they make decisions? Do children get in trouble if they make a wrong choice? Are children able to work through problems on their own?

The following self-assessment can help you look at the decision-making skills you model for children. You don't need to write out answers to these questions. Just be honest with yourself. Remember, there is no one "right" way to behave, but what you learn from this self-assessment may help you do some things differently.

Self-Assessment: Decision Making at Home

As a parent, do you:

- Think your children will make good choices as they grow up?
- Let children know that adults make mistakes?
- Ask children for help in making decisions?
- Make some decisions together as a family (for example, where to vacation or how to celebrate a birthday)?
- Think children see you as a strong decision maker?
- Offer children choices so they can make decisions?
- Help children understand the consequences of their decisions?
- Think your children make good decisions?
- Help children if they are unhappy with their decisions?
- Understand how peer pressure may affect children's decisions?

Watch Out For...

- Criticizing children for making bad decisions.
- Telling children they can't make a decision because they don't know how.
- Worrying about how children will react to your decisions.

Communication

Dear Family:

Communication is part of everyday life. Even infants communicate by crying and smiling. Preschool children may ask for a glass of juice, comment on the day or talk to a friend. Older students communicate about their studies and their daily lives.

Good communication skills open the door to learning about others and to expressing our own feelings. Talking and listening to children helps them learn how to communicate. Many communication skills are learned at home. Think about the communication skills you want your children to have. Do you model and practice these skills?

This self-assessment helps you look at the communication skills you model. You don't need to write out answers to these questions. Just be honest with yourself. Remember, there is no one "right" way to behave, but what you learn from this self-assessment may help you do some things differently.

Self-Assessment: Communication at Home

As a parent, do you:

- Let children hear you talking to other adults?
- Think what children say is important?
- Talk often with your children's teachers about school activities and how your children are doing?
- Teach children to express their anger in ways that don't hurt themselves or others?
- Ask questions about your children's day every day?
- Understand what children are talking about?
- Have family discussions, perhaps around the dinner table?
- Spend one-on-one time daily with your children (for example, reading to them)?
- Think your children can talk to you about their problems?
- Give clear directions when you ask children to clean the kitchen or put away toys?
- Enjoy listening to children talk to their friends?
- Ask questions that require more than yes or no answers?
- Teach children how to write thank-you notes or talk on the telephone?
- Laugh with children instead of at them?
- Let children cry when they need to?

Watch Out For...

- Making fun of children.
- Scolding children for crying.
- Discounting children's feelings.

Discipline

Dear Family:

As children learn how to handle stress, make decisions, solve problems and communicate, they will make mistakes. There are two ways of dealing with children when they make mistakes. We can punish them, or we can let them experience the consequences of their actions.

Discipline and guidelines help children know where the boundaries are. When children experience the consequences of their actions, they can learn from their mistakes.

Think about how you discipline children. Does your family help its members learn to be responsible? If you look into the future, do you think your grandchildren will grow up to be responsible, as they learn from your children what you are modeling today?

This self-assessment can help you set family guidelines about discipline. You don't need to write out answers to these questions. Just be honest with yourself. Remember, there is no one "right" way to behave, but what you learn from this self-assessment may help you do some things differently.

Self-Assessment: Discipline at Home

As a parent, do you:

- Expect children to be courteous, respectful and responsible?
- Speak clearly when you give children directions?
- Have clear and consistent rules so children know what is expected?
- Give children regular family jobs to do?
- Notice both good and bad behavior?
- Think your children are well behaved?

Watch Out For...

- Making threats you don't mean.
- Yelling before you think about what you're saying.
- Punishing instead of letting children experience the consequences of their actions.
- Using punishment that doesn't relate to the behavior (for example, not letting a child play with friends because she left her backpack at school).
- Making fun of children when they make mistakes.

Safety Habits

Dear Family:

Good safety habits help protect children from injury. The attitudes and habits you have about safety are noticed by children. Think about your safety habits. What are children learning from you? Think about what children learn when you install a smoke detector in your home or insist on using crosswalks and waiting for the light to change.

You don't need to write out answers to these questions. Just be honest with yourself. Remember, there is no one "right" way to behave, but what you learn from this self-assessment may help you do some things differently.

Self-Assessment: Safety Habits at Home

As a parent, do you:

- Think about safety each day?
- Teach your children the emergency numbers to call and post them for all family members to see?
- Teach children to be safe in the kitchen by taking safe actions yourself (for example, using knives correctly, keeping pan handles turned away from the edge of the stove, being careful with hot oils, watching children as they cook for themselves, carrying hot dishes correctly)?
- Give baby sitters information about safety?
- Keep stairways free of clutter?
- Store dangerous chemicals safely?
- Use reflective material on backpacks and clothing used in the dark?
- Know if your children follow rules for pedestrian safety (cross at crosswalks, walk on sidewalks, use crossing guards, etc.)?
- Know if the playground at your children's school is safe?
- Know if your children's school has a safety committee?
- Know what kinds of injury prevention skills are taught at your children's school?

Watch Out For...

- Ignoring safety rules "just this once."
- Thinking that "it won't happen to me."
- Criticizing other parents for being safety conscious.

(continued)

- Taking unsafe actions (such as standing on the kitchen counter to reach something).
- Overloading electrical outlets.
- Being "too busy" to fix unsafe things around your home.
- Asking children to wear protective items such as safety belts or bicycle helmets but not wearing them yourself.
- Teasing children about the way they look in safety equipment.
- Criticizing the school for requiring safety equipment.

Driving Safely

Dear Family:

Automobile crashes are a major cause of injuries and death. Children must learn to behave safely in the car. Adults can model these safe behaviors as they show children that they respect and obey the rules for safe driving and being safe in the car.

Children see your driving habits every time they get in the car with you. Are you a safe driver? Do you need to improve what you model for children?

The following self-assessment can help you think about how you model safe behaviors in the car. You don't need to write out answers to these questions. Just be honest with yourself. Remember, there is no one "right" way to behave, but what you learn from this self-assessment may help you do some things differently.

Self-Assessment: Driving Safely

As a parent, do you:

- Always wear your safety belt and insist that children wear theirs?
- Check the safety of your car?
- Obey the speed limit and follow basic rules of the road?
- Show respect for the work that police and highway patrol officers do to keep roadways safe?
- Allow joggers or bicyclists plenty of room on the road?
- Never drive after drinking and refuse to ride with anyone who does?

Watch Out For...

- Making negative comments about how others drive.
- Criticizing others for driving at the speed limit.
- Taking risks while you drive (for example, driving too fast, passing on the shoulder).
- Saying things such as "Uh oh, there's a cop. I'd better slow down."

Safety in Sports and Recreation

Dear Family:

As you take part in sports and recreation activities, you model for children the importance of a regular fitness program. You also model some important safety behaviors. Think about the behaviors you model during your recreational and sporting activities. Do children see you following important safety principles?

You don't need to write out answers to these questions. Just be honest with yourself. Remember, there is no one "right" way to behave, but what you learn from this self-assessment may help you do some things differently

Self-Assessment: Recreational Safety

As a parent, do you:

■ Think about the kind of clothing you wear when exercising?

■ Know how to swim?

■ Take care of your exercise and recreation equipment?

■ Know how to check equipment such as bicycles or ski bindings for safety?

■ Know if your children know how to take care of their sports equipment (bicycles, roller skates, skis, etc.)?

■ Make sure children wear life jackets when boating and wear one yourself?

■ Make sure children have the right clothing and equipment for sports and other activities?

■ Ask for help to provide safety equipment such as headgear for baseball players or bicycle helmets for bike riders?

Fire Safety

Dear Family:

Fire is a major cause of death and injury of young children. Ask yourself, "How conscious of fire safety am I, as a rule?" The following self-assessment can help you think about how aware you are of fire safety.

You don't need to write out answers to these questions. Just be honest with yourself. Remember, there is no one "right" way to behave, but what you learn from this self-assessment may help you do some things differently.

Self-Assessment: Fire Safety at Home

As a parent, do you:

- Have a smoke detector in your home and check it often?
- Keep flammable materials in a safe place, away from furnaces or other dangerous things?
- Know when your home heating system was last checked?
- Know when your chimney was last cleaned?
- Keep fire extinguishers in your home and car and know how to use them?
- Have regular fire drills at your home?
- Have a family escape plan so everyone knows how to get out of the home during a fire?
- Know the number to call in case of fire?

Watch Out For...

- Throwing trash into the fireplace.
- Using a piece of paper to ignite a pilot light.
- Thinking you don't need a smoke detector because you'll never have a fire.
- Leaving matches out where children can reach them.
- Using a paper cup as an ashtray, if you smoke.
- Leaving burning cigarettes in the ashtray when you're finished with them, if you smoke.

First Aid

Dear Family:

The need for first aid often arises when dealing with children. Adults should know what to do when minor injuries occur. They should also be careful to react quickly and calmly. When children see that you are calm, they will be less likely to panic. You can let children see that emergencies can be taken care of and teach them how to get help.

These questions can help you look at how you model first-aid habits. You don't need to write out answers to these questions. Just be honest with yourself. Remember, there is no one "right" way to behave, but what you learn from this self-assessment may help you do some things differently.

Self-Assessment: First Aid at Home

As a parent, do you:

- Have a first-aid kit in the home?
- Know what to do in an emergency?
- Know how to clean wounds to prevent infection?
- Know how to do cardiopulmonary resuscitation (CPR)?

Watch Out For...

- Telling children they are "accident-prone"—even if you think they are.
- Children who panic when they scrape a knee or cut a finger. (Why do they act this way?)
- Telling children they look funny or ugly when they have a bruise, scratch or cut.
- Telling children that it's babyish to cry when they fall or get hurt.

Personal Safety

Dear Family:

Experts estimate that one out of four girls and one out of eleven boys are sexually abused. The average age of a victim of sexual abuse is six to eight years old.

Abuse has to be explained carefully. Most children will not be abused, and we don't want children to lose their trust in most adults. But children need to learn that sometimes they have the right to protect themselves even when adults are around.

You can show children that their personal safety is important to you. Set a standard that shows respect for everyone's right to be in charge of her or his own body and the right to say no. You can also model ways to say no.

This self-assessment helps you look at how you model personal safety. You don't need to write out answers to these questions. Just be honest with yourself. Remember, there is no one "right" way to behave, but what you learn from this self-assessment may help you do some things differently.

Self-Assessment: Personal Safety at Home

As a parent, do you:

- Think children trust you with their problems?
- Know when children are upset and help them talk about it?
- Listen to children when they express anger, sadness or other emotions?
- Think your children know what to do if someone tries to abuse them (physically or sexually)?
- Talk with children about personal safety issues (including physical and sexual abuse)?

Daily Health Habits

Dear Family:

Children can learn many daily personal health habits that help prevent or control disease, such as washing hands and brushing teeth, at a very young age. When you wash your hands before eating, you give children a valuable lesson on hand washing. When you encourage children to brush their teeth, you let children know that this health habit is important.

You can become more aware of the health habits you model for children. Ask yourself, "What do my children learn from me about personal habits for staying healthy?"

You don't need to write out answers to these questions. Just be honest with yourself. Remember, there is no one "right" way to behave, but what you learn from this self-assessment may help you do some things differently.

Self-Assessment: Family Health Habits

As a parent, do you:

- Think you set a good example by your daily health habits?
- Let children often see you wash your hands?
- Encourage children to wash their hands before meals?
- Let children know you go to a dentist?
- See that children get regular dental check-ups?
- Encourage children to brush their teeth often and well?
- Try to keep household surfaces germ free?
- Make sure that children have all the recommended immunizations?
- Show children how to limit the spread of germs after sneezing and coughing?

Watch Out For...

- Criticizing others for their health habits.
- Telling children that they take too much time to wash their hands, brush their teeth or take a shower.

References

Bean, R. 1992. *The four conditions of self-esteem: A new approach for elementary and middle schools.* Santa Cruz, CA: ETR Associates.

Cohen, W. S. 1992. The role of the federal government in promoting health through the schools: Opening statement of Senator William S. Cohen. *Journal of School Health* 62 (4): 126-127.

Henderson, A. C. 1993. *Healthy schools, healthy futures: The case for improving school environment.* Santa Cruz, CA: ETR Associates.

Ikeda, J., and P. Naworski. 1992. *Am I fat? Helping young children accept differences in body size.* Santa Cruz, CA: ETR Associates.

Kane, W. M. 1993. *Step by step to comprehensive school health: The program planning guide.* Santa Cruz, CA: ETR Associates.

Mann, Horace. 1840. *On the Art of Teaching.*

National Commission on the Role of the School and the Community in Improving Adolescent Health. 1990. *Code blue: Uniting for healthier youth.* Alexandria, VA: National Association of State Boards of Education.

Seibert, D., J. C. Drolet and J. V. Fetro. 1993. *Are you sad too? Helping children deal with loss and death.* Santa Cruz, CA: ETR Associates.

Snider, M. 1990. Panel wants junk food off school plates. *USA Today,* 6 December, 1990.

U.S. Department of Health and Human Services. 1988. *National Center for*

Health Statistics: Annual report. Washington, DC.

U.S. Department of Health and Human Services, Public Health Service. 1991. *Healthy people 2000: National health promotion and disease prevention objectives.* DHHS Publication No. (PHS) 91-50212. Washington, DC.